YOU Are the New Prescription

Simple Shifts. Real Health. Lasting Change.

RAJA RAMASWAMY, MD

WITH

RANI RAMASWAMY, MD

YOU Are the New Prescription
© 2025 Raja Ramaswamy, MD

All rights reserved. No part of this publication may be reproduced, stored in a retrieval system, or transmitted in any form or by any means, electronic, mechanical, photocopying, recording, or otherwise without the prior written permission of the publisher, except in the case of brief quotations used in reviews or scholarly articles.

ISBNs
Paperback: 979-8-9988114-0-1
Hardcover: 979-8-9988114-1-8
eBook: 979-8-9988114-2-5

Published by Milari Press
Carmel, Indiana
Printed in the United States of America

Cover design by Sole at Luna Design
First Edition

For more information, visit www.rajaramaswamy.com

DEDICATION

We wholeheartedly dedicate this book to our parents, Rama and Padma, whose relentless work ethic and unwavering belief in us paved the way for where we are today. Their lives are a testament to the enduring power of sacrifice: they set aside their own dreams to provide a foundation from which we could pursue our aspirations.

To our spouses, Hillary and Nirdhar, whose unwavering love and support have been our greatest source of strength. Your belief in us and in this journey has made all the difference, and we are forever grateful.

And to our children Ari, Mila, Sahana, Eshan, and Saavan whose limitless joy and curiosity inspire us and give deeper meaning to our journey. You are the heart of our motivation, and we dedicate to you not only this work, but every step of our shared path. We are profoundly grateful for the love, laughter, and purpose you bring to our lives.

To all our readers and supporters, thank you for joining us on this journey.

ACKNOWLEDGMENTS

Thank you to Becky Alexander for her thoughtful developmental editing and to Lisa Guest for her meticulous copy editing. I'm also grateful to the late Rahul Desikan, MD, PhD, whose drive and expansive thinking left a lasting impression on how I approach the bigger picture. I want to acknowledge Joey Tiwari, MD, for his involvement in shaping the direction of the book. I'm also thankful to the patients and colleagues whose stories and experiences inspired what's written here.

A Word About Your Health

This book is meant to inform and inspire, but it's not a replacement for medical advice. Everyone's health is different, and what works for one person may not work for another. Please talk to your doctor or a trusted healthcare provider about any questions or decisions related to your health or your family's well-being.

"Go as far as you can see; when you get there, you'll be able to see farther."

— **Thomas Carlyle**

TABLE OF CONTENTS

Dedication iii

Acknowledgments iv

Part I: The Foundation — Building a Stronger You

Introduction: How Quickly Life Can Change 3

Chapter 1: Understanding Mental Health: Nurturing Your Inner Strength 9

Chapter 2: Mindfulness: Being Present in the Moment 31

Chapter 3: The Brain: Mastering Your Mind's Potential 45

Part II: The Body in Balance — Physical Health That Lasts

Chapter 4: Heart Health: Keeping Your Heart from Being a Time Bomb 73

Chapter 5: Vital Vessels: Ensuring Healthy Circulation 87

Chapter 6: Breaking Free of Unhealthy Habits: You Can Be a Healthier You 101

Part III: Whole Health for Everyone

Chapter 7: The Power of Prevention: Building a Healthier Tomorrow 145

Chapter 8: Health for All Women: Addressing Our Unique Needs and Maintaining Long-Term Wellness 169

Chapter 9: Health for All Men: Recognizing the Barriers that Keep Us from Seeking Help 191

Chapter 10: The Next Generation: Giving Our Children a Healthy Start on a Healthy Life 211

Chapter 11: After You Close the Book: Living Your Healthiest Life 235

Part IV: Tools to Take with YOU

Appendix A 241

Appendix B 242

Appendix C 245

Appendix D 246

Bibliography 247

About the Authors 261

PART I

THE FOUNDATION — BUILDING A STRONGER YOU

INTRODUCTION
HOW QUICKLY LIFE CAN CHANGE

Life was pretty simple when I was 17. My days were mostly about school and hanging out with friends. But everything changed when we found out my dad needed heart surgery....

One evening, after he'd attended a party, my dad felt a tightness in his chest, but it went away pretty quickly. Even though the pain subsided, he decided to visit the doctor soon after, a decision that probably saved his life. The doctor discovered his heart was in bad shape. The blood vessels were almost completely blocked, and Dad needed critical surgery right away.

We all knew heart disease was common in our family, but my dad had never shown any signs. That bomb had been ticking inside him without any of us knowing. At first, I didn't want to believe Dad's heart surgery was actually happening, but the reality and my fear hit me hard as they took him into surgery. Seeing him cry for the first time and then seeing my mom, my sister, and myself crying, too was something I'll never forget. I was scared.

My dad hadn't been very healthy. He didn't exercise much, and he didn't eat well. While he was in surgery, I couldn't stop thinking about what would happen if we lost him. The possibility was real, and I worried about how I'd take care of my mom and sister. I knew I'd need to grow up fast.

The surgery took six long hours. The doctors said it was touch and go, but my dad made it through. Seeing him after the surgery, all swollen and with tubes everywhere, was also scary. He looked so different. Although his recovery took time, within six months he was able to run a 5K an incredible milestone given the seriousness of his surgery. Our family life was never quite the same afterward, but many of those changes turned out to be good. We became closer as a family, learned to prioritize healthy eating, and began exercising regularly together.

That whole experience changed all four of us. We started talking more openly about how to care for our hearts and stay healthy. I realized how important it is for me to look after my own health, so I won't have to go through what my dad did. Dad's sudden and unexpected heart surgery also showed us how quickly life can change and how vital it is to take care of ourselves and those we love.

Making Positive Changes

Right away we started paying more attention to what we ate, making sure we had more fruits and vegetables on our plates. My dad started walking every day, a big change from before. We all learned a lot about heart health and how important it is to take care of ourselves. This new way of life wasn't easy at first, but seeing my dad get stronger made us want to keep going. We transformed our kitchen, swapping processed foods for whole grains and lean proteins, and restructured our family time to include more physical activities like hiking and cycling.

Talking about what happened with my dad also helped us grow closer as a family. Before his surgery, we didn't really talk about serious matters like our health or our feelings. But after seeing how quickly things can go wrong, we started to open up more to one another. We shared our fears as well as our hopes for the future. I also realized how precious time is and how we need to take care of each other. Now I think a lot about my own health and about making good choices. I want to be there for my wife and children the way my mother, my sister, and I were there for my dad.

This new lifestyle not only brought us closer to each other, but it also led to our greater involvement in our community. We started participating in local health drives and charity runs, and soon those activities were part of our new routine. Seeing my dad cross the finish line at his first 5K run, only six months after his surgery, was one of the most emotional moments I'd ever experienced. That milestone wasn't just about the distance my dad had run; it was about the fact that he had faced a life-threatening challenge and come out stronger.

As I moved into adulthood, the lessons I learned from that pivotal year stayed with me. I chose a career in health advocacy, driven by a desire to educate others about the importance of heart health. The memory of my dad's struggle still fuels my passion for helping others avoid the same fate.

Our journey through heart disease taught us that while genetics may load the gun, lifestyle pulls the trigger. We learned that every meal, every step, and every health check could be the difference between a ticking time bomb and a healthy, vibrant life. We chose the latter, and it has made all the difference.

A Map for the Journey to Health

My dad's heart surgery prompted us as a family to make some wise decisions about our health. Maybe you want to make some lifestyle changes, but you're not sure where or how to start. The abundance of information available at our fingertips in just seconds, through social media and AI, can easily overwhelm and confuse. In a world overflowing with health advice, finding clear and straightforward paths to wellness can feel like searching for treasure without a map. *YOU Are the New Prescription* is designed to be that map, making health information simple, direct, and empowering.

As physicians with years of experience caring for patients, we wrote this book to help you take control of your health. Medical professionals and medication play critical roles, but the daily choices you make, what you eat, how you manage stress, and how active you are have a profound impact on how healthy you are. Our own journeys, both professional and personal, have shown us that lifestyle choices can be the most powerful medicine. True health is about feeling strong, energized, and in control of your well-being. Although we can't control everything about our health, we can definitely manage a lot, and even our small, intentional choices can create lasting change.

This book brings together years of research, experience, and practical strategies. We have studied the science, consulted with experts, and drawn from our own lives to provide you with guidance that is both credible and easy to apply. Each chapter presents useful insights in a way that's accessible and engaging.

Rather than using complicated medical jargon, we talk with you about important health concepts as if we're having a conversation over coffee. Health information should empower you, not overwhelm you.

Throughout this book, you may notice that we repeat certain ideas. That's because every aspect of health is connected to every other aspect of health. Mental and physical health work together. Your heart and circulation depend on the choices you make each day. The habits you build affect everything from your energy levels to your ability to avoid disease.

This book is filled with real-life stories, including scenes from our own, that show how making small and manageable changes can lead to significant improvements in our health. If we can do it, so can you.

One more thing. You aren't just reading a book. You are, we hope, stepping into a new way of understanding and caring for your health. *YOU Are the New Prescription* will show you how much power you have in shaping your health and your future. Let's dive in and discover how you can become your own best medicine.

Your Health, Your Prescription

Health isn't something a doctor can prescribe; it's something each one of us has to build every day. For too long, we've approached health as something to address only when problems arise. But the truth is, YOU are the new prescription and the exact prescription you need.

The power to shape your health is in your hands, and the key is understanding the core principles that drive long-term well-being. That's where The Ramaswamy Prescription comes in.

This simple science-backed framework makes health sustainable, effective, and actionable.

The 5 Pillars of The Ramaswamy Prescription

1. **Nourish:** Fuel Your Body for Optimal Health
   - The foundation for longevity starts with what you put into your body.
   - Whole foods, essential nutrients, and anti-inflammatory eating drive

performance and prevent disease.

- Supplements and strategic nutrition optimize energy, focus, and cellular health.

2. **Move:** Daily Motion Means Lifelong Vitality

    - Your body is designed to move, so daily activity is nonnegotiable.
    - Choose exercise routines that support strength, cardiovascular health, and longevity.
    - Integrate movement into your busy life.

3. **Recharge:** Master Sleep, Stress, and Recovery

    - Sleep is medicine, so learn how to get deeper, more restorative rest.
    - Understand and control the link between stress and chronic disease.
    - To reset your nervous system, harness the power of mindfulness, breath work, and relaxation techniques.

4. **Protect:** Practice Preventative Health and Build Long-Term Resilience

    - Routine screenings and lab work can mean early detection and staying ahead of disease.
    - Read about cutting-edge longevity strategies, from fasting to inflammation control.
    - Understand your body's key health markers and how to improve them.

5. **Break Free:** Eliminate Habits That Are Holding You Back

    - Learn the science behind quitting smoking, drinking an excessive amount of alcohol, being addicted to sugar, and subjecting yourself to almost constant digital overload.
    - Incorporate mental rewiring and behavioral techniques to break destructive cycles.
    - See how environment, accountability, and mindset drive long-term behavior change.

How This Framework Shapes the Book

Whether we're talking about heart health, mental well-being, breaking bad habits, or building a lifestyle that protects your long-term health, every chapter of this book connects back to the prescription. This five-pillar system offers a clear, structured approach to improving your health in a way that is effective and sustainable. By the end of this book, you'll be able to:

- Take control of your nutrition, movement, recovery, and mindset
- Break free from unhealthy cycles and build habits that last
- Use science-backed health strategies to increase longevity and vitality

Remember, you have the power to write your own health story. With every small step you take, you're choosing vitality over limitation, strength over struggle, and thriving over merely surviving. Let's begin this journey together, creating a future that's healthy, resilient, and uniquely yours.

Raja Ramaswamy and Rani Ramaswamy

CHAPTER 1

UNDERSTANDING MENTAL HEALTH:

NURTURING YOUR INNER STRENGTH

In a world that often prioritizes physical well-being and outward appearance, the significance of mental health is too often ignored. Yet understanding and nurturing our mental health is crucial to a balanced, fulfilling life. This chapter explores the critical importance of mental health, highlighting its impact on every aspect of our existence.

Mental health is the bedrock of our emotional, psychological, and social well-being. Every day it influences how we think, feel, and behave. Like the solid foundation of a sturdy house, good mental health underpins our experiences, resilience, and happiness.

A healthy mental state enables us to make choices, face challenges, and build relationships. It empowers us to communicate, empathize, and maintain healthy social interactions. Life inevitably brings challenges ranging from work stress to personal loss. Mental health provides the tools we need to cope with these challenges, allowing us to adapt, find solutions, and recover from setbacks.

In addition, the deep connection between our mind and body means that mental health is inseparable from physical health. Stress, anxiety, and depression can lead to a variety of physical health problems, including heart disease, weakened immune systems, and chronic pain. Conversely, good mental health can enhance physical health and prompt better lifestyle choices, higher energy levels, and improved overall health. So that's why this book starts with the topic of mental health.

Your Quality of Life

Investing in your mental health is investing in your quality of life. Mental well-being enriches your experiences, enhances your creativity, and contributes to your sense of purpose and fulfillment. Good mental health is also key to feeling happy and satisfied with life. It helps us appreciate the moment, find joy in small things, and navigate life's ups and downs with grace.

And all of us will encounter those challenges in life. A healthy and robust mental state fosters resilience, allowing us to bounce back from adversity. Good mental health also encourages personal growth, pushing us to learn, evolve, and expand our horizons.

We Need to Talk

In recent years, the world has seen a growing mental health crisis. The stress caused by the rising cost of living, and the loss of close-knit communities have all made mental health struggles more common. Suicide rates, especially among men, have increased, leaving families heartbroken and communities searching for answers.

In my own family, we lost our cousin Serena to suicide. A kind and intelligent woman, she took her own life when she was in her thirties. Her heartbreaking story provides a powerful and haunting reminder of both the silent battles many people face and the urgent human need to talk openly, be heard, and find support.

We too often keep quiet about mental health. We need to face this issue boldly and bravely because what we learn from these tragic stories of struggle may save someone else's life. Serena's story shows us how crucial it is to be aware of other people's mental health and to support them if they're struggling.

When we were growing up, though, we rarely talked about our feelings. Doing so would have revealed weakness or vulnerability. The implicit message was "Deal with it," whatever circumstances we were facing and whatever the weaknesses or vulnerabilities we were feeling. Maybe your family made that same message clear.

Many of us admired Serena: she was smart, caring, and seemingly unshakable. She did well in school and eventually became a respected dentist. To us, Serena was a source of joy and wisdom, and she was always a comforting presence. But underneath her capable, calm exterior, Serena was trapped between her own desires and the family's expectations.

In our culture, elders often guide our life decisions, especially when it came to marriage. But choosing to follow her heart, Serena married someone who didn't meet the family's expectations. This choice led to estrangement from the family, and she felt lonely for years. The family's disapproval created a growing distance, isolating Serena from the people she loved and needed the most.

After five long years, our family had a chance to reconnect with Serena. We visited her, hoping to revive the warm relationship we once shared. But the person we found was not the Serena we remembered. She was no longer the vibrant person we knew. The light in her eyes had dimmed, and her joyful laughter was gone. Her home, once a place of comfort, felt cold and unfamiliar, filled now with unresolved pain and loneliness.

Realizing that Serena was struggling deeply with her mental health filled us with sadness. Clearly, the strong and lively cousin we remembered was carrying burdens too heavy for her to bear alone. Yet, raised as we were, none of us had the tools we needed to talk about her struggles or offer her support.

Sadly, Serena's story didn't have the ending we hoped for. Her internal battle, which she fought mostly alone, ended with her taking her own life. This loss left our grief-stricken family with many unanswered questions: What if we'd seen the signs of her distress earlier? What if we'd broken the silence that surrounds the topic of mental health? What if we'd offered her the companionship, support, and love she needed?

Mental Health Disorders

For me, Serena's death served as a call to action: what would I do to help break down the barriers that keep people suffering silently and alone? Her story teaches that we must talk openly about mental health; create safe spaces where people can share their struggles without fear of judgment; reach out with compassion to those who might be suffering in silence as they fight a hidden internal battle; and offer understanding and support to those who find the courage to speak up.

So, in this chapter dedicated to Serena and her memory, I invite each of you to become an advocate for mental health. All of us can honor Serena's memory by being there for others in their times of need, reminding them that it's OK to not be OK and that rather than being a sign of weakness, asking for help is a sign of strength and a step of hope. When we commit to listening, supporting, and standing by those who are fighting hidden battles, we will make mental health a priority, no one will face life's darkest moments alone, and stories like Serena's can end not in tragedy but in healing and health.

Sadly, mental health issues affect millions of people worldwide. (The medical term *mental health disorder* refers to a condition that significantly disrupts a person's thoughts, feelings, mood, ability to relate to others, and daily functioning.) The following statistics reveal the scope of today's mental health crisis:

- Approximately 1 in 4 people globally will experience mental health issues at some point in life. Currently, around 450 million people suffer from a mental disorder, making it one of the leading contributors to poor physical health worldwide.

- A common mental disorder, depression affects more than 264 million people around the world. In addition to being highly prevalent, depression carries a high risk of increased illness and earlier death, increasing the likelihood of developing cardiovascular and metabolic diseases by 40%.

- Anxiety disorders are the most common mental health condition in the United States, affecting 40 million adults, or 18.1% of the population, each year. Anxiety is a feeling of worry, nervousness, or fear about something that might happen, all of which are normal responses to stress. But when these feelings intensify, become constant, and interfere with daily life, they may be indicative of an anxiety disorder.

- Severe mental illness (SMI) affects about 5.2% of adults in the US each year, significantly interfering with or limiting one or more major life activities.
- Bipolar disorder impacts approximately 45 million people worldwide. Characterized by episodes of mania and depression, this disorder can significantly impair people's ability to function and impact their quality of life.
- Affecting more than 20 million people globally, schizophrenia is a severe mental disorder that disrupts how a person thinks, feels, and behaves. It can be incapacitating if left untreated.
- Eating disorders, such as anorexia nervosa and bulimia nervosa, affect at least 9% of the population worldwide. These disorders have one of the highest mortality rates among mental illnesses, underscoring their severity.

Occasional periods of stress or sadness are part of life, but persistent stress or sadness may point to a mental health disorder that often requires professional medical intervention or care.

Demographics of Mental Health

Mental health disorders impact men and women as well as specific age groups differently. Women, for instance, are more likely than men to experience depression and anxiety. In fact, women are almost twice as likely as men to be diagnosed with depression. This higher rate may be influenced by such factors as hormonal differences, societal roles, and the likelihood of seeking medical care. Additionally, in contrast to men, women are generally more likely to talk about their mental health struggles and seek professional help, which could lead to their higher rate of diagnosis.

Mental health disorders affect individuals across all age groups, but the prevalence of certain disorders can vary significantly:

- Children and Adolescents: In the US approximately 1 in 6 young people aged 6 through 17 are diagnosed with a mental health disorder each year, and the actual number may be even higher. Some research done in educational settings suggests that many cases go unrecognized or undiagnosed due to either the stigma attached to mental health issues or the lack of access to care.

- Young Adults: Among college students in the US, 1 in 3 reports having experienced significant depression, and nearly half have experienced overwhelming anxiety. Considering the pressures and challenges young adults face during this transitional life stage, the number may be higher. Once again, depression and anxiety disorders may not always be formally diagnosed or reported.

- Older Adults: About 15% of adults aged 60 and over suffer from a mental health disorder. This age group may also be underdiagnosed due to the general awareness that mental health decline is a normal part of aging

Why Mental Health Matters for Everyone

Although taking care of our mental health is crucial for our personal well-being, it's also important to recognize that mental health issues collectively have a significant impact on society as a whole. For example, depression and anxiety don't just affect how we feel; they also affect our ability to work and be productive. Globally, the economy loses about $1 trillion each year because of reduced productivity caused by these common mental health conditions.

In the US alone, serious mental illness results in $193.2 billion in lost earnings every year. When employees struggle with unresolved depression, they are 35% less productive, impacting not only their own lives but also the businesses they work for. On top of this, people with mental health disorders often face higher medical expenses, adding financial strain to their already challenging situation.

Clearly, investing in mental health is about individual well-being, and creating a healthier, more productive society. By prioritizing mental health, we can reduce the country's economic losses and improve the quality of life for everyone.

Access to Treatment

Despite the widespread nature of mental health issues, access to treatment remains limited. On average, only 44% of adults with a diagnosable mental health problem receive treatment. For children, the situation is even more concerning, with only about 50% of those aged 8 to 15 receiving the mental health support they need. In low- and middle-income countries, between 76% and 85% of the people with mental disorders receive no treatment for their condition. Several barriers contribute to the lack of access to treatment, including the stigma surrounding mental illness, the limited availability of mental healthcare professionals, the high cost of care when it is available, and an inadequate mental health infrastructure. The urgent need for improved access to mental health services will not be easily resolved.

Breaking the Silence

Although our world is gradually becoming more aware of mental health issues, the stigma remains. Many people don't talk about their mental health struggles because they fear being judged. They know that a segment of the population regards a mental health issue as a sign of personal weakness, a character flaw, or even a lack of the willpower needed to overcome difficulties, but this is simply not the case. Still, that fear contributes to men over the age of 50, like my uncle Raj, being among the least likely people to seek help for mental health issues.

Always the strong, silent type, Raj never talked about his feelings even when his struggle became obvious to those around him. Only after his passing did we learn he had been battling severe depression. The fear of people's judgment, rejection, and misunderstanding often leads individuals like my uncle to hide their suffering, making them less likely to seek help. Without support or treatment, mental health conditions can escalate. Such isolation can delay treatment, affect all aspects of life, worsen outcomes, and, in some cases, lead tragically to suicide.

Breaking Down the Stigma Attached to Mental Health

- Breaking down the stigma attached to mental health requires a multifaceted approach that involves education, open conversations, and promoting stories that humanize the struggle.
- **Education and Awareness:** Increasing public understanding about

mental health can challenge myths and change attitudes. Educational campaigns that provide clear facts about mental health are crucial. But personal education is necessary as well: do you know the signs of depression or anxiety in yourself or others? Taking the time to learn about the indications of mental health issues can make a big difference in how you perceive those issues. For example, recognizing that irritability or withdrawal in a friend may signal depression can prompt you to offer compassionate support rather than dismissing the behavior as simply being unfriendly or distant. Understanding these signs fosters empathy, encouraging a more supportive response toward mental health challenges.

- **Open Conversations:** Encouraging open discussions about mental health, whether in schools, workplaces, or families, can destigmatize these issues and create a more supportive environment for the people among us who are suffering. Younger people who post on social media are leading the way in this movement to normalize discussions about mental health. Many share their experiences openly, creating communities where others feel safe to do the same. But these conversations need to happen in real life as well, not only in online spaces. How often do you check in with your friends or family members to see how they're really doing?

- **Promoting Help-Seeking Behavior:** Society must champion the truth that seeking help is a strength, not a weakness. Have you ever hesitated to seek help because you felt that doing so was a sign of failure? We need to change that mindset. Highlighting accessible resources and celebrating those who take steps to improve their mental health can inspire others to do the same. Think about a time when you yourself reached out for help. What did you find empowering about taking that step?

- **Support Systems:** Building robust support systems, both formally through mental health services and informally through community support groups, can provide a safety net for people in need. Young adults, especially on social media, are doing a great job of creating online support networks where they share resources, advice, and encouragement. However, social media isn't the only avenue. Community groups, whether in person or online, also offer invaluable support. Do you have a support system you can rely on, or are you part of a more formal group that offers such support?

Breaking down the barriers that keep us from acknowledging and addressing mental health issues is not only a task for society at large; it's an effort that each of us can and ideally will be involved in. By educating ourselves, starting conversations, and being part of a supportive community, we can help create a world where mental health receives the care and attention it deserves.

Each of us can help to break down the stigma surrounding mental health. By being careful about our language, extending compassion, and supporting people around us, we can together help to create a society where no one feels they have to hide their struggles; where seeking help is applauded, not shamed; and where mental health is approached with the same seriousness and care as physical health.

After all, our mental health and our physical health are intertwined: each significantly influences the other. Chronic physical conditions can, for instance, increase the risk of developing mental health issues. An ongoing battle with illness or injury can take a toll on one's mental health, leading to increased risks of depression, anxiety, and emotional distress. The daily challenges, limitations, and stress of managing physical limitations can significantly affect one's psychological and emotional state.

Likewise, poor mental health can predispose individuals to physical health problems. Persistent stress, anxiety, or depression may lead to physical health issues like heart disease, high blood pressure, weakened immune function, and obesity. When constantly activated, our physiological response to stress wears down the body, making it more susceptible to illness.

Aisha Finds Her Calm

> Aisha, a 28-year-old single mom, was frayed from her retail job and raising two kids. Sleepless and snappy, she hit a low after crying alone one night. A friend urged her to see a counselor at a community center, who diagnosed anxiety. Aisha started weekly therapy on a sliding-scale fee, journaled her feelings nightly, and joined a free yoga class at the library. Three months later, she slept through the night, argued less, and laughed with her kids again. Asking for help wasn't giving up...it was her comeback.

Lifestyle Choices

Exercise, nutrition, sleep, and substance use not only affect our physical health but also have implications for our mental well-being.

- Regular physical activity is a powerful mood booster, reducing symptoms of depression and anxiety while simultaneously improving physical health.
- Nutrition significantly impacts brain function and mood, and a healthy diet supports mental well-being as effectively as it does physical health.
- Good quality sleep is essential for both mental and physical health. Poor sleep can make mental health issues worse and lead to physical problems.
- The use of, for instance, alcohol or marijuana as a coping mechanism for mental health struggles will harm both mental and physical health over time.

As we'll explore in the chapters ahead, understanding and optimizing our lifestyle choices can lead to significant improvements in our overall well-being.

Emotional Hygiene

Despite the fact that we sustain psychological injuries far more often than physical ones, we largely neglect the vital practice of emotional hygiene in our families and our schools. Emotional hygiene, the establishment and maintenance of emotional health, involves proactively managing and nurturing our psychological health. Just as we care for our physical bodies to prevent illness, we need to care for our minds to prevent psychological distress. We need to recognize and find healing for emotional pain stemming from loneliness, failure, rejection, and negativity, to name a few sources. Since experiencing these feelings can be painful, no wonder the common advice is to "Shake it off" rather than "Seek healing." But this dismissive attitude toward emotional wounds can lead to deeper psychological issues, including depression and anxiety.

Loneliness

Although we are constantly connected through social media, phones, and the internet today, many people feel more isolated than ever. Loneliness is not limited to being physically alone. Loneliness is feeling emotionally and socially disconnected from others, and that feeling can arise even when you're surrounded by people or connected through technology. The resulting psychological wound affects how we see ourselves and the world around us. When we feel lonely, our thinking can become distorted, making us believe we are less valuable or less worthy of love and relationship.

Research consistently shows that loneliness is harmful to both our mental and physical health. People who experience chronic loneliness have a 14% higher risk of dying early, a risk comparable to the risk of smoking cigarettes. Loneliness can also lead to high blood pressure, increased cholesterol levels, and a weakened immune system, making it harder for our bodies to fight off illnesses.

In a society where we might feel connected digitally, we must recognize the ongoing importance of real-life, meaningful relationships and invest in them. Understanding the dangers of loneliness and finding ways to connect with people on a deeper level can help protect both our mental and physical health.

Resilience

Coping with failure is another crucial aspect of emotional hygiene. If, after we fail at something, we convince ourselves that we are incapable of succeeding at anything, we might give up on life's challenges too soon or not try at all. Too many of us operate below our true potential because a single failure convinced us that we can't succeed. This mindset stunts growth and learning, preventing us from reaching our full potential.

Strategies for Emotional Hygiene

What does all this talk about emotional health mean for you? Have you ever felt low, been anxious, or found yourself struggling, but kept it to yourself because you thought it was better to soldier on? Do you have people you can talk to when you're not feeling your best? Or do you find it difficult to open up to others?

Those questions are intended to help you acknowledge how much time and effort you do or don't invest in your mental health. What specific steps can you take to improve your emotional health and hygiene? Here are some key strategies to try:

- **Check In with Yourself**: Set aside a few minutes each day to consider how you're feeling. If you're stressed, anxious, or feeling down, acknowledge those emotions without judging yourself.

- **Stop Emotional Bleeding**: Just as you clean a cut to prevent infection, it's important to address emotional wounds when they occur. You might seek support, extending to yourself the kind of compassion you would extend to a friend. Work, too, on challenging negative thoughts that are lodged in your mind.

- **Build Emotional Resilience**: Resilience helps us bounce back from setbacks. We set the stage for emotional resilience when we have realistic expectations, view failures as opportunities for growth, and maintain a positive outlook.

- **Foster Connections**: Combat loneliness by actively working to build and maintain strong relationships. Being open, vulnerable, and genuinely interested in others can strengthen your social network so it serves as a buffer in times of emotional distress. Taking time to connect with a friend or family member can also boost your mood.

- **Challenge Negative Self-Talk**: Pay attention to your inner dialogue. Challenge and replace negative thoughts with realistic and more positive ones. Doing so can boost your self-confidence and reduce the impact of failure.

- **Practice Mindfulness**: Staying connected with the present moment reduces stress and enhances emotional well-being. Regular practice of this mindfulness can improve your response to emotional challenges.

If you notice a loved one struggling, encourage that person to talk with you about what they're going through. Your willingness to listen without interrupting or offering solutions can be an incredible gift to that person. Sometimes, simply knowing that someone cares can make all the difference.

Improving Your Mental Strength

Mental strength is about harnessing the power of your mind to deal with the adversity you encounter; to overcome obstacles that arise; and to pursue your goals despite the fear of failure or rejection. Everyone can increase their mental strength with practice and perseverance, and understanding the nature of mental strength is the first step toward unlocking its power in your life. The key components of mental strength are:

- **Emotional Intelligence**: The ability to understand and manage your emotions positively in order to relieve stress, communicate effectively, empathize with others, overcome challenges, and defuse conflict

- **Grit**: A strong will to persevere toward long-term goals, choosing to maintain your effort and interest over the months and even years despite failure, adversity, and plateaus along the way

- **Optimism**: The practice of focusing on the positive aspects of every situation and expecting good things to happen, a focus that can lead you to take actions that increase the likelihood of positive outcomes

- **Mindfulness:** The quality of being present and fully engaged in whatever you're doing at the moment free from distraction, not judging yourself, and being aware of your thoughts and feelings without getting caught up in them. To practice mindfulness, start by focusing on your breath. Take a few deep breaths, paying attention to how the air feels as it enters and leaves your body. If your mind starts to wander, gently bring your focus back to your breathing. You can also practice mindfulness during daily activities, like eating or walking, by paying closer attention to the sights and sounds around you and to the sensations you're experiencing. Stay in the moment and observe your thoughts and feelings without letting them take over.

Developing mental strength requires dedication and self-reflection. The following strategies will help you build and then harness your mental resilience when you need it:

- **Challenge Yourself Regularly:** Stepping out of your comfort zone and taking on new challenges will strengthen your mental muscles and build your confidence in your abilities. You might, for example, travel to a new place, even if only to a nearby town you've never explored. The experience of successfully navigating unfamiliar surroundings can boost your confidence and adaptability. Or join a new class, whether it's a fitness class, an art workshop, or a public speaking course.

Learning something new not only challenges your mind but also provides opportunities to meet new people and gain fresh perspectives.

- **Develop a Growth Mindset**: Know that you can increase your abilities and sharpen your intelligence with effort, learning, and persistence. So embrace challenges, persevere despite setbacks, consider effort as the path to mastery, learn from criticism, and find lessons and inspiration in the success of others. If, for instance, you're struggling to learn a new skill like playing a musical instrument or learning a language a growth mindset encourages you to view the challenge as an opportunity to improve and grow. Instead of thinking, "I can't do this," try thinking, "I can't do this yet, but with practice, I will."

- **Extend Compassion to Yourself**: Be kind to yourself when you're experiencing pain or have failed at something. Recognize that imperfection is part of being human and give yourself grace during difficult times.

- **Build a Support System:** Surround yourself with people who encourage you. These supportive friends, colleagues, and teammates not only help in tough times but also make life more fun and enjoyable.

- **Focus on What You Can Control:** Rather than worrying, spend your energy on thinking helpful thoughts and acting on factors within your control, factors like your own reactions, your decisions, and the effort you invest in pursuing your goals. By focusing on what you can impact, you empower yourself to make positive changes, and you'll probably enjoy greater peace of mind.

- **Embrace Positive Habits**: Incorporate regular exercise, adequate sleep, healthy eating, and mindfulness into your routine. These habits not only improve physical health but also strengthen mental resilience.

- **Reflect on Past Successes**: When facing a new challenge, remind yourself of obstacles you've overcome in the past. This remembering can boost your confidence.

Social Media and Mental Health

Social media offers incredible opportunities to connect with other people and to access information instantly. However, it also presents challenges that can negatively impact our mental health. The constant exposure to carefully curated images and posts can, for example, lead to intensified feelings of inadequacy, greater anxiety, poor sleep, and depression. We can too easily fall into the trap of comparing our life to the highlight reels we see. It's not uncommon to feel that our accomplishments or experiences aren't enough when we compare them to what other people post. This sense of being "less than" can chip away at your self-esteem and make you feel pressured to present a perfect image of your life just to keep up with the people you see social media. Nearly half of today's teens feel overwhelmed by the pressure to gain likes and comments, evidence that the pursuit of online validation can lead to emotional stress.

The irony is that while social media is meant to connect us to one another, it can actually contribute to feelings of loneliness and isolation. Scrolling through posts and engaging in superficial interactions online too rarely provide the kind of deep, meaningful connections we human beings need. Those shallow exchanges can also rob us of time we might invest in real-life relationships and face-to-face interactions, leaving us feeling more disconnected than ever. In addition, digital overload can heighten anxiety and stress by disrupting sleep patterns, especially among young adults, and by contributing to a constant sense of FOMO (Fear Of Missing Out).

One of my best friends, Alex realized her constant scrolling was affecting her mental health. She decided to try a digital detox, starting with one weekend free from social media. During this time, she focused on activities she enjoyed, like hiking and spending time with family. The break helped her feel more connected to the people around her and less stressed about keeping up online. Inspired by this initial experience, Sarah now limits her social media use to 30 minutes a day, and she says that doing so has significantly improved her mood and overall well-being.

What's Your Plan?

So what steps might you take to protect your mental health yet still enjoy the benefits of social media? Start by recognizing when social media is making you feel worse instead of better. If you find that spending time online leaves you feeling drained or anxious, it might be time for a digital detox. Try setting aside a day or even a few hours to step away from your screens and focus on real-life interactions and activities. Limiting your social media use to 30 minutes a day has been shown to reduce feelings of loneliness and depression, leading to greater life satisfaction.

Be intentional and wise about your approach to social media. By setting healthy boundaries and being aware of how social media affects your mood and your thinking, you can enjoy staying connected without compromising your mental well-being.

10 Ways to Strengthen and Optimize Your Mental Health

1. **Think of Your Mental Health as Your Most Valuable Investment**

You wouldn't skip an appointment with your cardiologist or ignore a broken bone, so why overlook your mental well-being? Treat your mental health as an asset that appreciates over time. Whether you choose therapy, mindfulness, or setting boundaries, prioritize caring for your mental health in the same way you would prioritize setting up a retirement fund.

2. **Balance Mental and Physical Health Like a Pro**

Your mind and body work best when they are in sync. Swap one gym session a week for a mindfulness exercise, a walk in nature, or even a yoga class. Strengthening your body is important; so is giving your mind a break from the daily grind.

3. **Practice Emotional Hygiene Every Day**

Just like regularly brushing your teeth, take time regularly to check in with yourself. Are you carrying unnecessary stress? Holding on to resentment? A single deep breath, a journaling session, or even pausing for a moment can help you both let go of emotional clutter and do a reset.

4. **Unlock Your Brain's Natural Feel-Good Pharmacy**

Movement is medicine because exercise releases endorphins that instantly boost your mood. You don't need to train for a marathon to enjoy that boost. Twenty to 30 minutes of simple walking, stretching, or dancing to your favorite song can make a huge difference.

5. **Hydrate for a Sharper, Calmer Mind**

Feeling foggy or irritable? Dehydration may be the reason. Water fuels brain function, regulates mood, and keeps your stress level in check. So always have a reusable water bottle near your workspace and make hydration a daily habit.

6. **Upgrade Your Daily Routine with Small Mental-Health Wins**

Some of the best improvements to our life come from small daily choices. Step outside for five minutes of fresh air. Swap ten minutes of scrolling for some deep breathing. Pick one small action each day and let it snowball into lasting emotional health.

7. Take Control of Social Media Instead of Letting It Control You

Constant scrolling prompts comparison, lots of comparison, and adds stress as you see so many ways *you feel like* you don't measure up. Try establishing one phone-free day per week. Or maybe start by taking an hourlong break from social media before bed. And remember that social media is a highlight reel; it is *not* real life.

8. Get Outside and Let Nature Work Its Magic

Sunlight increases serotonin levels, making you feel happier and more energized. So step outside, even for a few minutes, and take a deep breath. Also, green spaces have proven to reduce stress, lower anxiety, and boost focus.

9. Surround Yourself with People Who Lift You Up

The people you spend time with affect your mental health. So choose to be around people who bring you joy, make you laugh, and support your well-being. Laughter is real medicine: it reduces stress and boosts happiness.

10. Give Your Mind the Rest It Deserves

Burnout doesn't come from working hard. It comes from never stopping. Put mental reset days on your calendar just as you would schedule a business meeting. Have a slow morning, unplug from technology, and/or spend an afternoon doing something you love. Your brain needs time to recharge.

Bonus Tip: Make Tending to Your Mental Health a Habit

Mental health is not something you fix once and forget about; it is a lifelong practice. Start by making one small change today and build from there. A healthier, happier mind results from consistent, intentional choices.

Your Action Plan for Mental Health

Reading about mental health is one thing, but real change only happens when you apply what you learn. This section can help you take action and start seeing results in your daily life.

Run a Mental Health Audit

Take a moment to check in with yourself. On a scale of 1 to 10, with 1 being "Help! I'm going under!" and 10 being "I've never felt better!", rate your current level of mental clarity, stress, and emotional well-being. Write down what is draining you and what is energizing you. What small changes could shift the balance and earn you a higher rating on the scale?

Select a Mental Health Nonnegotiable

Choose one small daily habit to make a nonnegotiable part of your mental wellness routine. Consider, for instance, five minutes of deep breathing, a morning entry in a gratitude journal, or an evening walk without distractions. Pick something simple and commit to doing it for the next seven days.

Try the 2-Hour Digital Detox Challenge

One day this week, put your phone on airplane mode for at least two hours. Use those two hours for something nourishing. Read, move, or simply sit in stillness. Then notice how you feel afterward. What shift in your mood happened when you stepped away from constant notifications?

Take a People Inventory

Who are the five people you spend the most time with? List the names and, next to each, your answers to these questions:

- Does this person uplift and inspire me?
- Do I feel drained after spending time with them?

- Do they support my well-being or add to my stress?
- Now take one small action to increase time with the positive influences—and be sure to set boundaries on the draining ones.

Make Time for a Mental Reset

Pick a reset activity that helps you recharge. Maybe it's journaling, a solo walk in nature, cooking a meal from scratch, or listening to music with your eyes closed. Schedule this into your week as you would an important meeting. If you don't give your mind a break, it will take one for you and that's called burnout.

Follow the One-Laugh-a-Day Rule

Laughter is scientifically proven to reduce stress and boost happiness. For the next seven days, make it your goal to laugh at least once a day. Watch a funny Instagram reel, call a friend who makes you laugh, or find humor in everyday moments. Notice how even a little laughter can improve your mood.

Practice the Five-Second Pause

Before reacting to stress, frustration, or anxiety, pause for five seconds and take a deep breath. Ask yourself, *Is this matter worth the cost of my peace?* Making this five-second pause a habit can, over time, rewire your response to stress.

Get Outside and Move

Every day for the next week, step outside for at least 10 minutes during daylight hours. Let the sun hit your skin. If possible, move your body while you're out there. Those 10 minutes can improve mood, regulate sleep, and lower stress.

Track Your Mood for a Week or Two

At the end of each day, jot down one word that describes how you felt that day. After a week, look for a pattern. What did your best days have in common? What made the tough ones harder? Use these insights to adjust your daily habits in ways that support your mental health.

Pick One and Start Now

Reading this list is great, but what will you do right now? Choose at least one action to put into practice today. Improving mental health is not about making drastic changes. Improved mental health comes with consistent, intentional choices that make a difference over time.

CHAPTER 2

MINDFULNESS:

BEING PRESENT IN THE MOMENT

Four years old and full of life, my daughter, Mila, was trying to show me something.

"Daddy, look at me! Watch my dance!" she called out, her voice filled with pure joy.

I was too busy with my phone to notice at first. Engrossed in the latest news, I gave her a distracted nod and a half-hearted "That's great, sweetie."

The screen had captured my attention, each swipe bringing a new flood of information. The constant stream of notifications, messages, and social media posts consumed me. Distracted by and engrossed in this digital chaos, I was oblivious to the real world around me.

When I finally looked up and saw Mila dancing all by herself, something inside me clicked. The contrast between her joy and my distraction hit hard. Mila's laughter had been filling the room while I was lost in a sea of far less important information. I felt a wave of guilt for choosing my phone over these precious moments with her. Clearly, I needed to make some changes.

I put my phone away and really focused on her. "Show me your dance again, Mila," I said, my voice expressing my genuine interest. I clumsily mimicked her steps, and she giggled at my attempts. This time her beautiful laughter filled my heart. With that sweet point of connection, I appreciated to a greater degree both the present moment and the precious human being right in front of me.

From this point on, I promised myself, *I will be more present, free from digital distractions and able to celebrate these little moments with Mila and my family*. So now every evening after dinner, we dance together. Her little hands guide me through the steps, transforming our living room into a magical place of connection and love.

Reflecting on what I was scrolling through on my phone before that epiphany, I realized it was mostly useless information and mind-numbing content. The hours I spent diving into the endless cycle of notifications, social media updates, and online chatter about current events contributed little to my well-being. Scrolling on my phone had become a habit that consumed valuable time that I could be spending with loved ones or engaging in other life-giving activities.

Maybe you've experienced this kind of "Aha!" moment. If so, know that you and I aren't the only ones who have been sucked in to screen time. The average person spends about 4 hours and 25 minutes on their phone each day. That time which all of us could share with friends, spend in the refreshing beauty of nature, or use to invest in our health and happiness adds up to more than two months every year!

That realization was eye-opening. It spurred me to not only limit my screen time but also to become more selective about the content I do consume. What value did each app or website add to my life? Did it bring joy or knowledge? If not, it wasn't worth my time. Instead, I opted to fill my days with enriching experiences: reading books, going for walks, playing games with Mila, and having unhurried, heartfelt conversations with my wife.

Slowly, I began to break free from the grip of mindless scrolling, and I rediscovered the delight of being fully present with those people I cherish most. Mila's dance had been a catalyst for this transformation. Her innocent joy and, since then, our shared moments of connection have kept me focused on what truly matters. The digital world can never provide the kind of fulfillment I find in the real, tangible moments of love and presence with my family.

Introduction to Mindfulness

Mindfulness is about focusing on the present moment and, as you do so, calmly acknowledging and accepting your feelings, thoughts, and bodily sensations without making any judgments about what you notice. This practice a kind of meditation helps you become more aware of your experiences. In many ways, mindfulness is the exact opposite of mindlessly scrolling on our phone, an activity that fragments our attention and numbs our mind. Dating back thousands of years, across many different cultures, mindfulness helps us experience more fully the now.

Among the benefits of mindfulness are:

- A strengthened immune system
- Enhanced sleep quality
- Reduced stress and
- Increased positive emotions

Mindfulness actually changes the brain, increasing gray matter density in areas linked to learning, memory, the regulation of emotions, and empathy. It also helps us focus better by tuning out distractions and improving memory, attention skills, and decision-making abilities. Moreover, mindfulness cultivates compassion and altruism, enhancing relationships by making us more present, attentive, and empathetic when we're with people. With so many benefits, why aren't we all making mindfulness a healthy habit?

We can practice mindfulness in formal meditation sessions, or we can weave it into our daily activities. Both approaches encourage a shift toward living moment by moment with our full attention focused on what we're experiencing and with genuine appreciation for all that experience entails. This practice can profoundly impact our physical, psychological, and social well-being, a fact indicating the pivotal role mindfulness can play in today's fast-paced, often digitally saturated life.

If you're new to mindfulness, finding a class online or downloading a mindfulness app can be a great way to begin. Many resources offer guided sessions to help you learn the practice of mindfulness. You can also start with this simple mindfulness exercise right now:

Take a few minutes to sit quietly, close your eyes, and focus on your breath. Notice the sensation of the air entering and leaving your body. If your mind starts to wander, gently bring your focus back to your breathing.

You can do this simple practice anywhere and anytime, and it will always help you to connect to the present moment.

Mindfulness as Medicine

The practice of mindfulness has been shown to effectively reduce anxiety and depression, lower blood pressure, and improve sleep quality. It can also enhance our ability to manage chronic pain and contribute to an overall improvement in our quality of life.

Mindfulness may even slow down the skin's aging process by impacting telomeres (the protective ends of chromosomes) and thereby preserving cellular integrity. Imagine that something as simple as mindfulness might be better for you than the most expensive face cream!

Additionally, mindfulness has been shown to elevate one's mood by influencing brain activities associated with emotion, attention, and body awareness. Specific breathing exercises can activate those areas of the brain, enabling us to manage our thoughts and emotional states more effectively.

By promoting greater body awareness and sharpening the ability to notice both the positive and the negative consequences of one's choices, mindfulness practices can also encourage such healthier habits and lifestyle changes as an improved diet and increased physical activity.

As a doctor, I would love to prescribe mindfulness to all my patients. I can't do that, but I can encourage them and you to write your own prescription for 10 minutes of mindfulness a day. This small but consistent commitment can lead to significant health benefits, possibly even reducing the need for medications like antidepressants. Research shows that regular mindfulness practice can manage symptoms of depression naturally and reduce reliance on antidepressants.

The transformative potential of mindfulness is undeniable as it alleviates symptoms of stress and anxiety; fosters more meaningful engagement with life; contributes to a heightened sense of well-being; and enriches our experience of the present moment. The practice of mindfulness is a solid cornerstone of psychological health and personal development.

Let's Get Mindful

To incorporate mindfulness into your daily life and make it a lifelong practice, start with small, manageable steps and gradually build for yourself a routine of various exercises and activities that fits into your lifestyle. You can find a wealth of resources and communities available online to support you on this journey.

1. **Make Mindfulness a Daily Practice**: Think about actions you do regularly, like drinking a cup of coffee, brushing your teeth, or walking to work, and practice being fully present in those moments. Notice the rich aroma of your coffee, the wind's quiet rustling of the leaves in the trees around you, or the familiar sounds of your family getting ready for their day. These small observations can help anchor you in the present moment, making mindfulness a natural part of your daily life.

2. **Build a Personal Mindfulness Routine**: Set aside a specific time each day, even a few minutes, to practice mindfulness. Start with simple exercises like these:

    - Deep breathing: Take slow, deep breaths, and as you do so, focus on the sensation of filling your lungs with air and then gently releasing it. This exercise can help calm the mind and reduce stress.

    - Mindful eating: Pay close attention to the experience of eating. Notice the flavors, textures, and aromas of your food, and focus on savoring every bite.

    - Body scan meditation: In your mind, scan your body from head to toe. Pay attention to any sensations, any tension or pain, and you'll connect with your body and be able to release physical stress.

    - These simple exercises are effective ways to integrate mindfulness into your daily routine.

3. **Engage with Other People**: Numerous resources, such as community meditation groups, local mindfulness workshops, yoga

classes, online forums, and mindfulness retreats, are available to help guide your mindfulness practice. Engaging with others who are traveling a similar path can provide motivation, accountability, and a valuable sense of connection.

Digital Detox

Phones are designed to be addictive…and guest what…they are:

- Americans check their phones an average of 144 times a day.
- A notable 60% of Americans sleep with their phones next to their bed.
- In the event of a house fire or other major disaster, 82% of Americans would make sure to take their phone with them before evacuating.

These statistics show that too many of us are allowing technology to take up too much of our energy and time. We need our phones and technology, but are we letting them dominate too much of our life?

The constant notifications, the ongoing social media updates, and the endless flow of information make it challenging to disconnect even though we know it's good for our mental and physical health. This overinvolvement with technology can increase stress, shrink attention spans, and reduce a person's real-world social interactions. But not only is our well-being at stake. Our habits are also shaping the next generation.

As parents, caregivers, and role models, the way we interact with technology sets the standard for our children. When they see us constantly on our phones, they consider it normal behavior. If we don't set boundaries for ourselves, we'll struggle to teach them to do the same. Furthermore, children are incredibly perceptive: they notice when we're more engaged with a screen than with them. What we model about our relationship with technology can potentially lead to our children's screen addiction or social isolation. They are learning what we're living out in front of them.

To start living and modeling a healthier relationship with tech, we can implement tech-free times during key moments of the day, such as meals, family gatherings, or before bed. These times can be opportunities to connect with loved ones, engage in meaningful conversations, and fully experience the present moment. Encouraging activities that foster mindfulness and presence, such as meditation, spending time in nature, or pursuing hobbies like gardening, crafting, or reading, can also help reduce screen time and enhance well-being.

By taking these steps, not only are we improving our own relationship with technology, but we're also modeling healthy habits for our children. Demonstrating the value of real-world connections over virtual ones teaches them the importance of balance in an increasingly digital world. It's about showing them that while technology has its place, it should not dominate our lives. We can guide our children toward a future where they can enjoy the benefits of technology without becoming controlled by it.

So, as you work on reducing your own screen time, remember that you're paving the way for your children to do the same. By being present with them, prioritizing face-to-face interactions, and setting clear boundaries for phone use, you're helping them develop a healthier, more balanced approach to technology that will serve them well throughout their lives.

Emma's Moment of Peace

> Emma, a 35-year-old nurse, was unraveling from 12-hour shifts. At home, she'd scroll her phone, missing chats with her partner, and headaches piled on. A coworker's mindfulness tip sparked a change. Emma tried five-second pauses to calm her mind and banned phones during meals. After shifts, she stretched for 10 minutes with a free meditation app's music. Two months later, her headaches vanished, and she felt truly present. One night, she and her partner danced in the kitchen, giggling like kids. Those pauses were her reset button.

Cultivate Gratitude and Joy

Want an easy way to improve your mood? Cultivate gratitude and joy! In other words, recognize and appreciate the positives in life, and you'll notice improvements in your mood, attitude, and well-being. Looking for the positive in every situation, even in challenging ones, will help you see the positive.

Practicing gratitude can significantly improve your mental health. More specifically, fostering a positive mindset can counter the negativity bias many of us have. By *negativity bias*, I mean dwelling on the negative and overlooking the positive. When you focus on gratitude, you pay attention to what's good in your life, releasing in the brain happiness-inducing chemicals like serotonin and dopamine.

You can effectively cultivate gratitude by using mindfulness practices that emphasize being thankful for what you have. Let's try it now:

1. **Close your eyes and imagine a loved one at their happiest.** Picture that person's smile, replay their laughter in your mind, and think about the joy they bring into your life.

2. **Notice how this Step #1 affects your mind and body.** Do you feel your face relaxing? Are you smiling? Is a sense of warmth or calm spreading through your body? Pay attention to these physical manifestations of gratitude.

3. **Reflect on a recent positive experience.** Think of something good that happened to you recently, and it doesn't need to be particularly momentous. Maybe a colleague spoke a kind word to you, or you enjoyed a delicious meal or a moment of genuine laughter. How did this experience make you feel? Take a moment to appreciate it fully.

4. **Put your gratitude into words, speak them out loud, or, after you finish this exercise, write them down.** Acknowledging your gratitude verbally can deepen the positive impact on your emotions. You might even thank in writing or in a phone call the person who showed you kindness or brought you joy in some other way.

5. **Take a deep breath and slowly open your eyes.** As you exhale, be sure to hold onto this sense of gratitude and carry it with you into the rest of your day. Let it influence your interactions and your mindset.

Such practices don't take much time, but they can profoundly impact your well-being and happiness. The benefits of gratitude include better sleep, improved focus, higher self-esteem, and increased patience. Gratitude can also strengthen interpersonal connections and enhance the quality of your relationships as you tell people that you love and value them.

You might also end each day by thinking of three things you are grateful for. Again, they don't have to be remarkable. They can be as simple as a delicious meal, a friend's kindness, or the warmth of your bed. Reflecting on moments that prompt gratitude can help you drift off to sleep with a sense of contentment and peace.

In addition to thinking about what you're grateful for, reflect on what brings you joy. You know I find joy in dancing with my daughter. Those moments fill my heart with happiness. You might find joy in attending comedy events, bird watching, or hiking. Whatever it is, make time for this joy-giving activity. Prioritize whatever makes you smile and fills you with energy. Which of the activities that came to mind will you do this weekend? By regularly engaging in what brings you joy, you'll lift your mood and find additional reasons to be grateful.

10 Ways to Be More Present in the Moment

1. **Train Your Mind to Show Up**

Your mind loves to wander, but being present is a skill you can develop and strengthen. Start by learning to recognize throughout the day when you drift into overthinking, worrying, or checking out mentally. When you notice that drift, simply take a deep breath and return to whatever is happening right now.

2. **Reduce Phone Time; Increase Real-Life Time**

A smartphone is undoubtedly the biggest obstacle to living in the present. So try limiting how much time you spend on apps, put your phone in another room during meals, and/or schedule screen-free hours in your day. The less time you spend scrolling, the more time you'll have for what truly matters.

3. **Engage Your Senses to Help You Stay Grounded**

When you feel distracted, reconnect by tuning into what you can see, hear, smell, and feel. Notice the way sunlight warms your skin... the scent of the coffee in the morning... or the sound of laughter nearby. Presence starts with awareness.

4. **Give Others the Gift of Your Attention**

The best way to deepen relationships is to be fully present with the people in your life. Make eye contact, genuinely listen rather than planning what to say next, and resist the urge to check your phone mid-conversation. People know when you are truly there with them.

5. **Intentionally Focus on One Task at a Time**

Multitasking scatters your focus and increases stress. Instead, commit to doing one thing at a time. When you eat, just eat. When you work, focus on that task alone. When you listen to music, let yourself get lost in the sound. Doing less, but doing it fully, makes life richer.

6. **Take Strategic Breaks to Recharge**

Pushing through fatigue or stress doesn't make you more productive. Instead, it actually drains you. Step away from your screen, go for a walk, or simply sit quietly for a few minutes. A well-timed break resets your mind and helps you return to the task at hand with clarity.

7. **Pause Before Reacting to Emotions**

When stress, anger, or frustration arise, pause rather than react. Take a deep breath and give yourself a few moments to consider an appropriate response. This simple practice can help you calmly make wiser choices in any situation.

8. **Be Intentional about Your Breathing**

Your breathing can help anchor you in the present moment. If you're not convinced, take three slow, deep breaths right now and notice how your body relaxes. Practicing this throughout the day will bring you back to the present whenever you feel scattered.

9. **Come Up with Your Own Version of Meditation**

You can meditate not only when you're sitting silent and still but also while you're taking a walk, painting, or even cooking. The goal is to quiet your mind so you can fully engage in the experience. Find ways to meditate that help you slow down and tune in.

10. **Find Magic in the Ordinary**

Staying present comes with appreciating the small things like a kind smile, the sound of rain, the fragrance of your morning coffee. Pay attention to the moments you usually overlook, and you'll start to see beauty everywhere.

Your Action Plan for Being Present in the Moment

Being present is not something you do naturally; you *train* your mind to embrace the present moment. The more you practice, the easier mindfulness becomes. The following exercises can help you establish mindfulness in your everyday life.

1. How Present Are You?

On a scale of 1 to 10, how present do you tend to be in your daily life?

- Do you often find yourself distracted, multitasking, or stuck in your head?
- When was the last time you had an in-person conversation without checking your phone?
- How often do you fully enjoy small moments like drinking your coffee or feeling the sun on your skin?

Write down your score and then, next to it, one **step you can take today** to start improving it.

2. The One-Minute Awareness Reset

For **one minute**, stop what you are doing and do the following instead:

- Close your eyes and take a deep breath.
- Listen to the sounds around you.
- Notice the feeling of your feet on the ground.
- Attend to any thoughts that come up without judging them.

How do you feel after that one minute? If you can reset in a single minute, imagine what 10 minutes of awareness would do for you.

3. The One-Thing-at-a-Time Experiment

For the next 24 hours, commit to **doing one thing at a time.**

- When you eat, just eat.
- When you talk to someone, focus fully on that person.
- When you work, turn off notifications and work.

Notice how it feels when you slow down and give each task your full attention. Does your stress level change? Do you feel more in control of your time?

4. Your Personalized Ritual for Being Present

What is one **simple ritual** you can add to your day to bring yourself back to the present moment? Here are some suggestions:

- Take three deep breaths before starting a new task.
- Drink your coffee and enjoy it instead of checking emails while you sip.
- Do a quick stretch before you pick up your phone in the morning.

Write down whatever ritual you choose and commit to doing it every day this week.

CHAPTER 3

THE BRAIN:

MASTERING YOUR MIND'S POTENTIAL

Emma woke up to the sound of her alarm, but instead of feeling rested and ready to start the day, she was overwhelmed by a sense of fatigue, the kind of bone-deep tiredness that sleep doesn't fix. She hit snooze a few times, hoping for a few more moments of peace before facing the day. But during those extra minutes intended for rest, her mind spun with worries and a dull sense of dread about what the day would hold.

Eventually, Emma dragged herself out of bed, each movement slower and more demanding than the last. As she stood in front of the mirror brushing her teeth, she barely recognized the person staring back at her. Her face looked pale except for the dark circles under her eyes. She used to enjoy her morning routine, taking time to do her makeup and choose an outfit she liked. But lately she found herself throwing on whatever was clean, unable to muster the energy to care.

Sitting at the kitchen table, Emma stared blankly at her cup of coffee. She usually loved the rich aroma and comforting warmth, but now this once-special morning ritual felt like another task, a chore to get through. Not feeling even a little hungry, she left her breakfast untouched, again skipping what was once a small pleasure. She couldn't shake the feeling that nothing really mattered. She didn't have the energy for the effort eating would require.

Her commute to work was a blur. Emma's mind was a foggy mess of worries and self-criticism. She couldn't shake the feeling that she was falling behind in every aspect of life. At work, for instance, tasks that had been quite manageable now seemed insurmountable. She felt like she was climbing a mountain and would never get to the peak. Her inbox was filled with emails she couldn't find the energy or clarity of thought to respond to, and she struggled to focus during meetings.

Her colleagues noticed the change. Once lively and full of ideas, Emma had become withdrawn and quiet. She politely declined invitations to lunch and after-work drinks. It wasn't that she didn't want to go, part of her longed for that human connection, but making conversation and pretending to be OK? Emma didn't think she could do it. She was living in a mental and emotional fog. She felt separated from the world by an invisible barrier that she couldn't break through.

As the day wore on, a knot of anxiety tightened in her chest. It was as if a weight were pressing down on her, making it hard to breathe. She tried to push through it and focus on her work, but the feelings were too strong. The doubts that plagued her mind were relentless: *Was she good enough? Was she letting everyone down?* The sadness that clung to her was like a shadow, following her everywhere, never letting up.

By the time she got home, Emma was utterly drained even though that morning she couldn't have imagined being any emptier than she was then. The idea of cooking dinner or even watching her favorite TV show had no appeal, which was fine because she had no energy. She collapsed onto the couch and scrolled mindlessly through her phone, but nothing held her attention. The messages from friends went unanswered. Even when they reached out, concerned about her absence and her silence, Emma didn't know how to explain what she was feeling. How could she when she didn't fully understand it herself?

That night, Emma lay in bed staring at the ceiling, replaying the day's events in her mind. She felt trapped in a cycle she couldn't break as every day blended into the next with no relief in sight. Her tears came slowly at first and then in waves as she realized how much she truly wanted things to change but didn't know where to start. She felt alone even though she knew she could reach out to any of a number of people who genuinely cared about her. The weight of her sadness was too much to bear. All she could do was hope that tomorrow would be different, though she feared it wouldn't be....

Emma's experience offers a window into the reality of depression, a condition that affects millions of people, altering the way they feel, think, and handle daily activities. Clinical depression isn't simply feeling sad: it's a deep, pervasive condition that can make even the simplest tasks seem overwhelming and leave a person feeling isolated and hopeless. Understanding depression is a crucial step in maintaining brain health and overall well-being. Mental health struggles are real but not insurmountable. Seeking help is essential to reclaiming one's life.

The Widespread Incidence of Depression

Depression is one of the most common mental health disorders, with the World Health Organization (WHO) estimating that more than 264 million people globally suffer from it. In the US alone, about 17.3 million adults experience at least one major depressive episode in any given year, according to the National Institute of Mental Health.

Symptoms of depression can include persistent sadness, loss of interest in activities once enjoyed, changes in appetite and sleep patterns, and difficulty concentrating or making decisions. In severe cases, depression can lead to thoughts of self-harm or suicide, a fact that underscores the critical need to understand the disorder and know when intervention is critical.

Strengthening Our Brains to Prevent and Combat Depression

Understanding how to work with our brains to manage depression is crucial. For some people, lifestyle changes such as regular exercise, a healthy diet, and sufficient sleep can make a significant difference. Exercise, for instance, releases endorphins, the natural chemicals in the brain that improve mood and relieve pain. Additionally, mindfulness and cognitive-behavioral therapy (often referred to as CBT) are effective tools for managing the negative thought patterns often associated with depression.

However, it's also important to recognize when something more than lifestyle changes might be needed. Depression is a complex condition that can have a biological basis, meaning that medication is necessary for some people. Antidepressants can help correct imbalances in brain chemicals that affect mood and emotions. For many, a combination of medication and therapy offers the best approach to managing depression.

When to Seek Help

So, how do we know when to seek help? It's important to listen to our body and our mind. If you or someone you know experiences persistent feelings of sadness or hopelessness or demonstrates a lack of interest in daily activities for more than two weeks, it's time to consider seeking professional help. Early intervention, before symptoms worsen, can make the journey to brain health easier and help restore a sense of normalcy sooner.

Remember, there's no shame in seeking help. Just as we wouldn't hesitate to go to the doctor for a broken bone or to take medicine for a physical ailment, we shouldn't shy away from getting the support we need for our mental health. Whether through therapy, medication, or a combination of both, taking action is a powerful step toward healing.

The Human Brain

The human brain is the most incredible organ in our bodies. It is responsible for every discovery, innovation, and creative project humanity has ever accomplished. It's the source of our joy, our happiness, and the wide range of emotions we feel, and it helps us solve problems and handle complex situations better than any other species can. Despite all its amazing abilities, the brain can also be affected by conditions that dramatically change our lives, making the brain both a source of potential vulnerabilities as well as our greatest strengths.

Astonishingly, the human brain accounts for only about 2% of our body weight but it demands 20% of the body's energy and caloric intake, a testament to its ceaseless activity and the heavy workload it carries. Each day, we make about 35,000 decisions, a statistic that demonstrates the brain's extraordinary ability to navigate life's challenges with astonishing speed and adaptability. It processes complex situations, understands intricate patterns, and devises innovative solutions, making it important not only for individual survival, but for the advancement of society as a whole. But its prowess extends beyond intellectual achievements; the human brain is also the wellspring of our emotions, of our joys, sorrows, and desires, allowing us to experience the richness of life in its fullest hues.

A brain's health is evident in mental clarity, emotional stability, a keen memory, and the ability to solve problems and think creatively. In contrast, signs of an unhealthy brain are persistent forgetfulness, difficulty concentrating, ongoing mood swings, and erratic behavior, any one of which may indicate stress, fatigue, or a more serious conditions like a neurodegenerative disease. Recognizing these signs helps us appreciate when our brain is functioning well and alerts us when we might consider seeking help.

Imagine your brain as a super powerful computer that's way smarter and more multifaceted than any machine ever built. This supercomputer works nonstop even when you're sleeping, making sure you keep breathing, your heart keeps beating, and you can dream.

But the brain does more than merely keep us alive. It's also the place where all our thoughts and feelings come from. It lets us enjoy our favorite songs, solve tricky puzzles, and feel love for our families and friends. But did you know that every time you learn something new, your brain changes a little bit? It's like adding a new book to a huge library full of knowledge. And just as muscles get stronger with exercise, your brain gets better the more you use it.

Nutrition: Fueling Your Brain with Healthy Foods

So what can we do to keep our brains healthy? The saying "you are what you eat" holds particularly true when it comes to brain health. The foods we consume have a profound impact on how our brains function, affecting everything from cognitive performance to emotional well-being. A balanced diet rich in specific nutrients can help protect against cognitive decline, improve memory, and boost overall brain function.

Essential Nutrients for Brain Health

1. **Omega-3 Fatty Acids:** Omega-3 fatty acids, particularly those found in salmon, mackerel, and sardines, are crucial for brain health. These healthy fats are vital components of brain cell membranes and have anti-inflammatory effects that can protect brain cells from damage. Omega-3s are also linked to improved cognitive function and memory as well as a lower risk of neurodegenerative diseases like Alzheimer's.

2. **Antioxidants:** Foods rich in antioxidants, such as berries, dark chocolate, and leafy greens, help protect the brain from oxidative stress that can damage cells and lead to cognitive decline. Antioxidants neutralize free radicals, those harmful molecules that can cause inflammation and damage brain cells. Including a variety of colorful fruits and vegetables in your diet ensures you get a wide range of these protective compounds.

3. **Vitamins and Minerals:**

    - **Vitamin E:** Found in nuts, seeds, and spinach, Vitamin E is an antioxidant that helps protect brain cells from damage. It's also been associated with a lower risk of cognitive decline.

    - **B Vitamins:** B vitamins, especially B6, B12, and folate, play a crucial role in brain health by helping to produce and maintain new brain cells and neurotransmitters. These vitamins are found in whole grains, eggs, and leafy greens.

    - **Magnesium:** This mineral, found in foods like almonds, spinach, and avocados, supports the brain's plasticity, which is essential for learning and memory.

4. **Whole Grains:** Whole grains like oats, barley, and quinoa are rich in the complex carbohydrates that provide a steady supply of glucose to the brain. The brain's primary source of energy, glucose also stabilizes blood sugar levels, helping us maintain focus and concentration.

5. **Hydration:** Staying well-hydrated is crucial for brain function. Even mild dehydration can impair attention, long-term memory, and mental processing speed. Drinking plenty of water throughout the day ensures that your brain stays sharp and functions optimally.

Brain-Boosting Foods to Include in Your Diet

- **Fatty Fish:** Rich in the omega-3s that are essential for brain function
- **Berries:** High in antioxidants that protect the brain from oxidative stress
- **Nuts and Seeds:** Provide healthy fats, antioxidants, and vitamins that support brain health
- **Leafy Greens:** Packed with vitamins like folate, which is important for cognitive function
- **Whole Grains:** Offer a steady release of glucose to keep your brain energized
- **Dark Chocolate:** Contains flavonoids, caffeine, and antioxidants that boost brain function

Sleep: The Brain's Maintenance System

Sleep is not only a time for physical rest; it is a crucial period when the brain undergoes vital processes that maintain its health and function. During sleep, the brain consolidates memories, clears out toxins, and repairs itself. Neglecting sleep can lead to a host of cognitive issues, including memory problems, impaired judgment, and an increased risk of neurodegenerative diseases.

The Importance of Sleep for Brain Health

1. **Memory Consolidation:** During sleep, the brain processes and then stores the information learned during the day, transferring it from short-term to long-term memory. This transfer process is essential for learning and retaining new information. Without adequate sleep, we can struggle to recall information and effectively perform cognitive tasks.
2. **Toxin Removal:** The brain's unique waste removal system known as the glymphatic system is most active during sleep. This system clears out harmful toxins, including the protein beta-amyloid that can build up and form plaques associated with Alzheimer's disease. Getting

enough sleep ensures that the brain can effectively clear out these toxins, reducing the risk of cognitive decline.

3. **Emotional Regulation:** Sleep plays a crucial role in regulating emotions. Lack of sleep can lead to increased irritability, stress, and anxiety that can negatively impact mental health. Chronic sleep deprivation has been linked to a higher risk of developing disorders like depression and anxiety.

4. **Cognitive Function:** Sufficient sleep is essential for maintaining attention, solving problems, and making decisions. Sleep-deprived individuals often struggle to concentrate, experience slower reaction times, and find critical thinking more difficult, all of which can impair both their performance of daily tasks and their ability to make decisions.

Tips for Improving Sleep Quality

- **Establish a Sleep Routine:** Go to bed and wake up at the same time every day, even on weekends, to regulate your body's internal clock.

- **Create a Relaxing Bedtime Routine:** Before bed, engage in calming activities like reading, taking a warm bath, or doing some relaxation exercises.

- **Limit Screen Time:** Exposure to blue light from screens can interfere with the production of melatonin, a hormone that regulates sleep. Try to avoid screens for at least an hour before bed.

- **Keep Your Sleep Environment Comfortable:** Be sure your bedroom is cool, quiet, and dark. Investing in a comfortable mattress and pillows can also make a significant difference in your sleep quality.

Be Mindful of Food and Drink: Avoid heavy meals, caffeine, and alcohol close to bedtime because they can disrupt sleep.

Mental Challenges: Exercise for the Brain

Just as physical exercise strengthens the body, mental challenges are crucial for keeping the brain strong and resilient. Engaging in activities that stimulate the brain helps maintain cognitive function, build new neural connections, and protect against age-related decline.

The Benefits of Mental Challenges

1. **Cognitive Resilience:** Engaging in mentally stimulating activities helps build cognitive reserve, which is the brain's ability to cope with damage and continue functioning well. Cognitive resilience is also crucial for delaying the onset of symptoms of neurodegenerative diseases like Alzheimer's.

2. **Neuroplasticity:** The brain has the remarkable ability to reorganize itself by forming new neural connections, a process known as neuroplasticity. Mental challenges such as learning a new skill or language encourage neuroplasticity, keeping the brain adaptable and able to continue learning throughout life.

3. **Memory Improvement:** Activities that challenge the brain, such as doing puzzles, playing strategy games, or acquiring new information, can enhance memory and recall abilities. Keeping the brain active and engaged is essential for maintaining memory function as we age.

4. **Problem-Solving Skills:** Mental challenges improve the brain's problem-solving abilities by encouraging logical thinking, creativity, and innovation. Regularly engaging in tasks that require critical thinking helps sharpen these skills that are vital for navigating daily life and making decisions.

Ideas for Mental Exercises

- **Puzzles and Brain Games:** Sudoku, crosswords, and memory games are great ways to challenge the brain and improve cognitive function.

- **Learning a New Language:** Language learning is a complex cognitive task that enhances memory, attention, and problem-solving skills.

- **Playing a Musical Instrument:** Music requires the brain to coordinate multiple tasks simultaneously, strengthening neural connections and improving cognitive abilities.

- **Reading and Writing:** Engaging with new information by reading or expressing thoughts by writing stimulates the brain and encourages critical thinking.
- **Strategy Games:** Games like chess or card games that require planning and strategy can help improve cognitive function and decision-making skills.

By incorporating into your daily routine these healthy habits, proper nutrition, adequate sleep, and regular mental challenges, you can support your brain's health and ensure it continues to function at its best. Taking care of your brain is about preventing disease, enhancing your quality of life, maintaining cognitive function, and enjoying a sharp, resilient mind throughout your days.

Neurological Disorders: When the Brain Doesn't Work as It Should

The human brain, with all its incredible capabilities, is also susceptible to a range of disorders that can have life-changing consequences. These conditions become greater concerns as we age, and many people fear the impact of brain disorders on their quality of life in later years. Whether it's the progressive memory loss of Alzheimer's, the debilitating tremors of Parkinson's, or the sudden devastation of a stroke, these disorders can profoundly affect our ability to live independently and enjoy our later years.

Given the significant impact that neurological disorders can have, it's no wonder that many of us are concerned about brain health as we age. The good news is, we can take steps today to improve our brain health and potentially reduce the risk of developing these conditions. A combination of a healthy diet, regular physical activity, mental challenges, and stress management can better our chances of maintaining a high quality of life well into our later years.

Here's a look at some of the most common neurological disorders and the number of people impacted worldwide:

- **Neurological disorders**, including strokes, brain injuries, and Alzheimer's disease, affect up to 1 billion people worldwide.
- **Dementia** affects approximately 50 million people globally, with this number expected to triple by 2050 due to aging populations.

- **Parkinson's disease** leads to progressive deterioration of motor functions and currently impacts more than 10 million people worldwide.

- **Epilepsy**, a prevalent neurological disorder that often means recurrent seizures, affects about 50 million people globally.

- **Multiple sclerosis (MS),** with symptoms ranging from mild numbness to severe disability, affects over 2.8 million people worldwide.

- **Stroke** is a leading cause of disability: Every year 15 million people suffer a stroke. Of these, 5 million die, and another 5 million are permanently disabled.

Neurological disorders are the leading cause of disability and the second leading cause of death globally. Stroke alone accounts for nearly 11% of total deaths worldwide. Similarly, brain conditions like Alzheimer's disease and other dementias rank as the seventh leading cause of death globally.

These statistics highlight the importance of being proactive about our brain health. Studies suggest, for example, that up to 35% of dementia cases are preventable through lifestyle changes. By adopting healthy habits now, we can improve our chances of living a fulfilling life free from neurological disease.

How Can We Reduce Our Risk?

Let's explore some specific ways to improve brain health and reduce the risk of neurological disorders:

1. Maintain a Brain-Healthy Diet

A balanced diet rich in nutrients is crucial for brain health. Diets like the Mediterranean and DASH (Dietary Approaches to Stop Hypertension) have been shown to reduce the risk of cognitive decline. These diets emphasize the following:

- **Healthy Fats**: Include sources of omega-3 fatty acids like fish, flaxseed, and walnuts that support brain cell structure and function.

- **Antioxidants**: Fruits, vegetables, and whole grains provide antioxidants that combat the oxidative stress that is linked to neurodegeneration.

- **B Vitamins**: Foods rich in B vitamins (like leafy greens, beans, and fortified cereals) help reduce levels of homocysteine, a compound associated with brain atrophy and dementia.

2. Engage in Regular Physical Activity

Physical activity is one of the most powerful tools for preserving brain health. Every week aim for at least 150 minutes of moderate-intensity exercise, such as brisk walking, swimming, or cycling. Exercise increases blood flow to the brain, supports the growth of new brain cells, and enhances cognitive function. Specific activities like aerobic exercise have been linked to larger hippocampal volume, the area of the brain involved in memory.

3. Avoid Tobacco and Limit Alcohol Use

Tobacco use is a major risk factor for stroke and other neurological disorders. Although perceived to be safer, e-cigarettes and vaping still pose risks to brain health, particularly due to nicotine's impact on brain plasticity. As soon as a person stops smoking, the risk for stroke and other neurological disorders decreases significantly, and benefits like improved circulation, better oxygen delivery to the brain, and a reduced risk of cognitive decline start to accrue.

When it comes to alcohol, moderation is key: no more than one drink per day for women and two for men. Excessive alcohol consumption can lead to brain shrinkage as well as increase the risk of dementia and other cognitive disorders. Reducing alcohol intake, especially binge drinking, can help preserve cognitive function as we age.

4. Manage Cardiovascular Health

Maintaining cardiovascular health is directly linked to brain health. High blood pressure, diabetes, and high cholesterol can all increase the risk of stroke and dementia. Here are three ways to manage these risks:

- **Monitor Blood Pressure**: Keep your blood pressure within a healthy range (below 120/80 mmHg).

- **Control Blood Sugar Levels**: To prevent damage to blood vessels in the brain, manage diabetes with proper diet, exercise, and, if needed, medications.

- **Manage Cholesterol**: Lowering LDL cholesterol through diet, exercise, and possibly medications can reduce the risk of brain damage caused by clogged arteries.

By making these lifestyle changes, you're not only improving your overall health but you're also actively reducing your risk of serious neurological conditions. These steps are an investment in your brain's future, offering the possibility of a longer, healthier life with a lower risk of cognitive decline.

In addition, key risk factors linked to dementia are hypertension, hearing loss, obesity, depression, diabetes, and social isolation. Taking steps to manage these risk factors could significantly reduce the likelihood of dementia. If you're dealing with any of these factors, talk to your doctor now about how to manage them effectively. Your doctor can provide guidance on medication, lifestyle changes, and other interventions that may help mitigate these risks.

Managing Key Risk Factors

Take a moment to recognize which of these key risk factors, if any, need your attention:

- **Hypertension**: Regularly monitor your blood pressure and discuss with your doctor if it's consistently high. Medications, a balanced diet, and regular exercise can help keep it in check.

- **Hearing Loss**: Hearing aids and other devices can significantly improve hearing, in turn reducing the cognitive load on your brain and helping you to maintain cognitive function.

- **Obesity**: A healthy diet and regular exercise are key to managing weight, and a healthy weight lowers the risk of diabetes and hypertension.

- **Depression**: Seek help if you experience symptoms of depression. Therapy, medication, and lifestyle changes can make a big difference in your mental health and reduce your risk of cognitive decline.

- **Diabetes**: Managing blood sugar levels through diet, exercise, and medication is crucial to preventing complications that can affect the brain.

Social Isolation: A Hidden Risk Factor

Social isolation is a significant but often overlooked factor contributing to dementia. Humans are inherently social beings, and regular interaction with other people is vital for mental health. Loneliness and a lack of social connections can lead to cognitive decline and increase a person's risk of developing dementia.

Practical Tips to Combat Social Isolation:
- **Stay Connected**: Yes, it takes time and energy, but maintain regular contact with friends and family. Even simple phone calls or video chats can help you feel connected.
- **Join Community Groups**: Get involved in community activities or join clubs that interest you. Whether you choose a book club, a gardening group, or a fitness class, staying socially active can stimulate your mind and reduce feelings of loneliness.
- **Volunteer**: Volunteering can provide you with a sense of purpose and connection. It's a great way to meet new people and stay engaged in your community.
- **Explore New Hobbies**: Trying out new activities can introduce you to new social circles and keep your brain active.

The Importance of Both Education and Early Intervention

Education plays a critical role in improving outcomes for people at risk of dementia. Being aware of public health campaigns and becoming educated about the signs and symptoms of brain disease can significantly improve both the chance of early diagnosis and the outcome of treatment, in the long run enhancing quality of life and reducing healthcare costs. Early intervention is key. Catching symptoms early may mean delaying the onset of severe symptoms and improving the effectiveness of treatments.

Proactively managing these risk factors, staying socially connected, and seeking early intervention can greatly contribute to maintaining brain health and reducing the risk of dementia. Remember, it's never too early or too late to start taking care of your brain health. Small changes today can lead to significant benefits in the future.

Common Brain Diseases

The human brain, while an organ of astounding complexity and capability, is also susceptible to a variety of diseases that can significantly impact health and quality of life. This section explores some of the most common brain diseases, their symptoms, and potential impact.

Alzheimer's Disease: Alzheimer's disease is the most common type of dementia, affecting memory, thinking, and behavior. Symptoms usually develop slowly and worsen over time, eventually becoming severe enough to interfere with daily tasks. Early signs include memory loss, particularly forgetting recently learned information; difficulty making plans or solving problems; trouble completing familiar tasks; getting confused about time or place; and changes in mood or personality. As the disease progresses, individuals may experience more severe memory loss, have difficulty recognizing loved ones, and experience significant changes in behavior and mood. Approximately 5.8 million Americans aged 65 and older live with Alzheimer's, with the number projected to rise to nearly 14 million by 2050.

Parkinson's Disease: Parkinson's is a progressive nervous system disorder that affects movement. Symptoms start gradually, sometimes starting with a barely noticeable tremor in one hand. Tremors are common, but the disorder also commonly causes stiffness or slowed movement. In the early stages of Parkinson's disease, a person's face may show little or no expression, and their arms may not swing when they walk. Speech may become soft or slurred. Symptoms worsen as the condition progresses over time.

Multiple Sclerosis (MS): This disease of the central nervous system can affect the brain and spinal cord, causing problems with vision, arm or leg movement, sensation, or balance. A lifelong condition that can sometimes cause serious disability, MS can occasionally be mild. The exact cause of MS is unknown, but it's considered an autoimmune disease in which the body's immune system attacks its own tissues.

Epilepsy: This central nervous system disorder causes brain activity to become abnormal, resulting in seizures, periods of unusual behavior or sensations, and sometimes loss of awareness. Anyone can develop epilepsy: it affects males and females of all races, ethnic backgrounds, and ages. Treatment with medications and sometimes surgery can control seizures for the majority of people with epilepsy.

Stroke: Every year strokes affect approximately 795,000 people in the United States alone, according to the Centers for Disease Control and Prevention (CDC). Globally, the World Health Organization estimates that strokes cause around 11% of total deaths, positioning it as the second leading cause of death in people aged 20 years and over. Beyond its immediate threat to life, a stroke can affect mobility, speech, and cognitive abilities and sometimes leave survivors facing significant disabilities. Up to 50% of stroke survivors suffer from lasting disabilities that severely impact their daily lives.

Research, however, suggests that up to 80% of strokes could be prevented through lifestyle changes and awareness. Key preventative measures include the following:

- Controlling high blood pressure (the leading cause of stroke)
- Managing heart disease
- Reducing cholesterol levels
- Maintaining a healthy weight
- Exercising regularly
- Not smoking
- Limiting alcohol consumption

Strive for a healthier lifestyle and schedule regular checkups with your doctor.

What Are the Signs of a Stroke?

Quick action can significantly reduce the severity of a stroke and improve the chances of survival. Individuals who receive treatment within three hours of their first symptoms often have less severe outcomes. The acronym FAST outlines the symptoms and protocol:

- Face drooping
- Arm weakness
- Speech difficulties
- Time to call emergency services

In summary, although the frequency of strokes is alarming, we do have ways to raise awareness and to prevent them. By knowing what puts a person at risk for a stroke and being able to recognize any warning signs in yourself, you can lower your chances of having one. Simply eating healthier, staying active, and keeping an eye on your blood pressure can reduce the long-term effects of strokes, help prevent strokes altogether, and even save lives. Reducing stress, getting enough sleep, and continuing to learn new things are all important for keeping your brain in top shape. These simple new habits can make a big difference in your overall health and in the quality of your life.

Evelyn Finds Her Rhythm

> Evelyn, a 62-year-old retired piano teacher, first noticed a subtle tremor in her left hand. At first, she thought maybe too much coffee. But when her handwriting began to shrink and she felt stiffness getting out of bed, she brought it up to her doctor. Tests confirmed early-stage Parkinson's.
>
> The diagnosis hit hard. Evelyn feared losing her independence and identity. But her neurologist offered a plan: medication to manage symptoms, but also lifestyle changes. Evelyn joined a Parkinson's support group, practiced daily hand stretches, and walked laps in her garden each morning to music. She even started boxing twice a week at a local gym, designed for patients like her.
>
> Six months in, her balance improved, and her tremors were steadier. More importantly, she felt emotionally stronger. She couldn't control the diagnosis but she could still write music, move her body, and stay connected. Parkinson's hadn't silenced her it just gave her a new rhythm.

Stress and Brain Health

Chronic stress can have profound implications for your brain health. Prolonged exposure to stress can lead to the deterioration of brain cells and the reduction of brain size, particularly affecting the areas responsible for memory and learning. The American Psychological Association notes that at some point, 77% of people in the US experience physical symptoms caused by stress. In addition, stress has been linked to several mental health issues, including depression and anxiety, highlighting the need for effective stress management strategies to protect brain health (National Institute of Mental Health).

Chronic stress triggers the release of cortisol, a hormone that, in high levels, can damage the hippocampus, the region of the brain crucial for forming new memories and for learning. The prefrontal cortex of individuals with high levels of chronic stress is reduced in volume, threatening the decision-making, emotional regulation, and social behavior that the prefrontal cortex guides. Long-term exposure to stress can also disrupt synaptic regulation, leading people to avoid interacting with others, and this isolation further exacerbates mental health issues.

Chronic stress is detrimental to physical health as well as mental health. Stress contributes to high blood pressure, heart disease, obesity, and diabetes. Stress-related hormonal changes can lead to inflammation, a known contributor to various chronic diseases, including neurodegenerative diseases like Alzheimer's.

Prolonged exposure to stress can impair such cognitive functions as attention, memory, and problem-solving skills. Stressed individuals often perform worse on cognitive tasks compared to their less stressed counterparts.

So how can we reduce our feelings of stress? The following practices have been shown to lower stress levels and promote mental well-being:

- Mindfulness
- Meditation
- Being in Relationship
- Adequate Sleep
- Lifelong Learning
- Exercise

Being in Relationship

Social support and strong interpersonal relationships protect against the negative effects of stress. Spending time with close friends or family, whether you share a meal, go for a walk, or simply talk about your day, can help you feel more connected and less isolated. Participating in social activities, joining a club, attending community events, volunteering in your community can also provide a sense of belonging and purpose, and that feeling significantly reduces stress. These interactions not only lift your mood but these experiences of positive emotions reduce the harmful effects of stress on body and mind.

Many people benefit from therapy: it provides them with a valuable opportunity to talk through challenges and gain new perspectives on their thoughts and behaviors. Cognitive-behavioral therapy (CBT) is a well-established approach that helps individuals identify and modify their stress-inducing thoughts and behaviors, thereby reducing the overall impact of stress on the brain. Through CBT, people learn practical strategies to manage their stress, improve their mental health, and develop healthier ways of thinking about and coping with life's difficulties.

The Importance of Sleep

As mentioned in the earlier discussion of dementia, sleep is a critical time for brain health and function, including a reduced sense of stress. During sleep, the brain engages in various processes, including consolidating memories, clearing out toxins, and repairing itself. According to the National Sleep Foundation, adults require between 7 and 9 hours of sleep per night, yet approximately one-third of American adults report that they usually get less than that recommended amount. Inadequate sleep can lead to cognitive decline, reduce a person's attention span, and impair one's ability to learn. Therefore, ensuring you get quality sleep in the recommended quantity is essential for maintaining your cognitive function and overall brain health.

Lifelong Learning as Brain Exercise

Learning something new is a workout for the brain that promotes the growth of new neural connections and enhances cognitive reserve. The concept of "use it or lose it" applies to brain function, with studies indicating that continued learning can help delay cognitive decline and reduce the risk of dementia. Engaging in intellectually stimulating activities also significantly reduces stress, as it provides a positive distraction, increases feelings of achievement, and promotes mental well-being. Activities like reading a book on a new topic, attending an evening class, learning to play a musical instrument, or taking up a new hobby not only keep your brain agile but also foster a sense of accomplishment and relaxation, counteracting the negative effects of chronic stress.

My friend Richard had ALS (amyotrophic lateral sclerosis, also called Lou Gehrig's disease), a condition that primarily affects motor functions. Despite his physical limitations, Richard's mental sharpness remained, a testament to the resilience of the human brain and the potential benefits of stress management, quality sleep, and continuous intellectual engagement. Taking care of your brain through stress management, quality sleep, and continuous learning can help you stay sharp and engaged, able to enjoy life to the fullest for as long as possible.

Physical Exercise

Physical exercise with its stress reduction benefit is not just beneficial for the body; it's also crucial for brain health. Regular physical activity can significantly reduce the risk of developing high cholesterol, hypertension, diabetes, and other conditions that impact brain function. The American Heart Association recommends at least 150 minutes of moderate-intensity aerobic exercise per week, an amount that improves cholesterol levels and lowers blood pressure, thereby significantly reducing the risk of stroke and heart disease by up to 20%. Furthermore, exercise enhances insulin sensitivity, which can prevent or help a person manage diabetes. According to the Alzheimer's Association, the absence of insulin sensitivity doubles an individual's risk of developing dementia. Finally, physical exercise also stimulates the release of chemicals in the brain that affect the health of brain cells, the growth of new blood vessels in the brain, and even the abundance and survival of new brain cells.

Smoking and Alcohol

Smoking and drinking don't always offer the stress reduction people may expect. Whatever initial relaxation those activities may offer, the reality is, smoking and excessive alcohol consumption are two lifestyle choices that significantly harm brain health. Smoking not only increases the risk of cardiovascular diseases but also accelerates cognitive decline. The World Health Organization reports that smokers have a 45% higher risk of developing dementia than nonsmokers.

Some researchers believe that moderate alcohol consumption, such as a glass of red wine, may have certain health benefits, but it's important to understand the risks associated with excessive drinking. The Centers for Disease Control and Prevention (CDC) defines heavy drinking as consuming 15 or more drinks per week for men and 8 or more for women. Chronic heavy drinking can lead to irreversible brain damage that impacts memory, decision-making, and impulse control.

But what exactly is "a drink?" A standard drink is typically 12 ounces of beer (5% alcohol content), 5 ounces of wine (12% alcohol content), or 1.5 ounces of distilled spirits or liquor (40% alcohol content). Understanding these measurements can help you keep track of your alcohol consumption and make healthier choices.

If you're concerned about your drinking habits, consider opting for low-alcohol beverages or mixing drinks with low-sugar sodas. (Avoid high-sugar alternatives like fruit juice because they can also have negative health impacts.) If you're finding it difficult to manage your alcohol intake, talking to a healthcare professional can provide valuable support and guidance.

The Power of Positivity

Individuals with a positive attitude toward aging and toward life in general are less likely to suffer from dementia and cognitive decline and more able to cope with stress. A positive outlook and emotional well-being really can bolster brain health, enhance your cognitive function, and build resilience against mental decline. Older adults who maintain a positive outlook on aging believing that they can remain active, healthy, and engaged as they grow older perform better on memory tests and are more likely to recover from disabilities than people who have negative ideas about getting older. The way we think about aging can have a real impact on our mental and physical health.

How can we develop a more positive mindset? Mindfulness and stress-reduction techniques are two options. Exercising regularly, avoiding harmful habits, and spending time with upbeat people also contribute to a positive mindset.

Regular physical activity, such as walking, swimming, or yoga, boosts blood flow to the brain, promotes the growth of new neurons, and helps reduce stress, all of which are vital for maintaining cognitive health. Avoiding harmful habits like smoking and excessive alcohol consumption protects the brain from damage and lowers the risk of conditions such as dementia and stroke.

So can practices that encourage gratitude and joy. Reflect every day on something you're thankful for. Maybe you're savoring a friend's act of kindness yesterday, today you appreciate the simple pleasure of a good meal, and tomorrow you may witness a beautiful sunset. Also make a point of engaging in activities that bring you joy, whatever those activities are. Know that doing these favorite activities for other people can amplify their benefits. For instance, volunteer to coach a sport you love, help others learn the kind of needlework you're passionate about, or contribute to your community by sharing your love for teaching in an afterschool tutoring program. In addition to activities like these, make the choice to see the world in a positive light. You'll improve both your mental well-being and your brain's ability to stay healthy and resilient.

By integrating regular exercise, healthy habits, and positive emotional practices into your daily routine, you're not only taking care of your body but you're also nurturing your mind, setting the stage for a life of vitality and fulfillment.

Taking a proactive approach to your brain health is essential. Regular physical exercise, avoiding harmful habits like smoking and excessive alcohol consumption, and fostering a positive emotional environment are all key to maintaining a healthy brain. These aren't just preventative measures; they're also crucial elements of living a fulfilling life. By adopting these practices, you can significantly reduce your risk of developing brain-related conditions and enhance your overall well-being.

What you can do today

Consider this call to action. Integrate one new habit into your routine whether it's dedicating a few more hours to restful sleep, picking up a book on a new subject, or taking a brisk walk daily and challenge yourself to reduce stress through mindfulness or meditation. Also, if you smoke, seek resources to help you quit. Remember, every positive choice you make is an investment in your brain's vitality and longevity. You have the power to improve your brain health, so act on that truth and ensure for yourself a brighter, healthier future.

10 Ways to Obtain Optimal Brain Health

1. **Turn Down Stress Before It Shrinks Your Brain**

Chronic stress floods your brain with cortisol, a chemical that can literally shrink your memory center. Try this: When stress spikes, pause to take five deep breaths or go for a 10-minute walk outside. Your brain will thank you.

2. **Treat Sleep Like a Brain Detox**

Sleep is your brain's cleaning crew. While you sleep, your brain flushes out toxins linked to memory loss and cognitive decline. Set a tech curfew for one hour before bed, dim the lights, and aim for between 7 and 9 hours of sleep.

3. **Challenge Your Brain Like You Challenge Your Muscles**

Your brain craves stimulation. Learning something new whether it is playing the piano, speaking Spanish, or solving puzzles creates new neural pathways that keep your mind sharp and flexible.

4. **Move Your Body, Feed Your Brain**

Exercise literally grows your brain. Just 30 minutes of movement increases blood flow, boosts memory, and protects against dementia. If the gym is not your thing, dance in your kitchen or take a brisk walk after lunch.

5. **Lower Your Blood Pressure, Protect Your Brain**

High blood pressure silently damages your brain, increasing your risk of stroke and memory loss. Check your numbers regularly, cut back on processed foods, and get moving. The goal? 120/80 mmHg or lower.

6. **Quit Smoking and Vaping Before Those Actions Shrink Your Brain**

Smoking accelerates your brain's aging and chokes off oxygen to brain cells. If quitting feels impossible, start small. You might delay your first cigarette by 30 minutes or swap vaping for deep breathing.

7. **Rethink Alcohol Before It Rethinks You**

Alcohol shrinks brain volume. If you drink, stick to one drink per day for women and two for men. Alcohol can cause slower thinking, a weaker memory, and an increased risk of dementia. You might also experiment with alcohol-free alternatives.

8. **Nourish Your Brain with Connection and Joy**

Loneliness is as bad for your brain as smoking is. So strengthen and/or expand your social circle, call an old friend, or get involved in activities that bring you joy. Your emotional health directly impacts your brain health.

9. **Protect Your Head Because Your Brain Has No Backup**

A single concussion can increase your risk of dementia. Wear a helmet when you're biking, use nightlights in your home to prevent falls, and work to maintain your balance as you age. A simple injury can have lifelong consequences.

10. **Train Your Brain to See the Good**

Negative thinking wires your brain for stress; gratitude rewires it for resilience. So before bed, write down three good things from your day. A grateful brain is a stronger, healthier brain.

Your Action Plan for Brain Health

Reading is great, but acting on what you read is what transforms your brain health. Use this section to apply what you've learned.

1. Brain Health Check-In

On a scale from 1 to 10, rate your brain health.

- Do you often feel mentally sluggish or forgetful?
- How much quality sleep do you get?
- Are you regularly exercising and eating brain-healthy foods?

Write down one area where you need improvement and commit to taking one small step today.

2. The 7-Day Brain Boost Challenge

For the next seven days, commit to one of the following practices:

- Get **7 to 9 hours** of sleep every night.
- Swap **one processed food** for a brain-boosting option like berries, nuts, or leafy greens.
- Take a **30-minute walk** or do a workout that gets your blood pumping.
- **Learn something new**: watch a documentary, read about a topic you know nothing about, or practice a new skill.
- Take **five deep breaths** to reduce stress.
- At the end of the week, reflect on how you feel. Do you feel sharper? More focused?

3. Your Personalized Brain Protection Plan

Pick one long-term habit to start developing today:

- Check your blood pressure on a regular basis
- Stop smoking
- Reduce your alcohol intake
- Make sleep a top priority

PART II

THE BODY IN BALANCE — PHYSICAL HEALTH THAT LASTS

CHAPTER 4

HEART HEALTH:
KEEPING YOUR HEART FROM BEING A TIME BOMB

If you read the opening chapter, you know that my father's heart was like a ticking time bomb. His heart disease had been completely unnoticed and therefore gone undiagnosed for too long.

If you don't take care of your heart, it may also become a time bomb that could explode anytime. If that hypothetical sounds scary, let its harsh truth compel you to not ignore your heart's health. After all, your heart keeps you alive by moving blood throughout your body, providing every part the oxygen and nutrients we need to keep going. Despite the heart's absolutely essential function, a lot of us forget to look after our hearts, and that neglect puts us in danger.

Does Heart Disease Run in Your Family?

In countries all around the world, heart disease is the number one cause of death. According to the World Health Organization, heart disease accounts for more than 17.9 million deaths annually, which is 31% of all global deaths. Among these, coronary heart disease and stroke claim the most lives. The Centers for Disease Control and Prevention (CDC) reports that in the United States, one person dies every 36 seconds from cardiovascular disease. These statistics aren't merely numbers; they represent millions of families affected by the loss or suffering of a loved one every year.

The increase in heart disease among younger populations is a troubling trend. This rise is largely driven by rising obesity rates, physical inactivity, and poor dietary habits. This shift also underscores the urgent need to reevaluate health education and establish age-appropriate preventative measures starting at a younger age.

If you have a history of heart disease in your family, you may understandably be concerned about your own risk. Don't hesitate to get your heart checked out. Start now to take proactive steps toward understanding and managing your heart health. Adopting healthier lifestyle choices, including a balanced diet, regular physical activity, and routine health checkups, can make a significant difference. By addressing these factors early, you'll help safeguard your future well-being and potentially reduce your risk of heart disease.

When I saw how heart disease affected my own family and learned how serious it can be, I knew I had to change how I lived. I didn't want to live scared; I wanted to enjoy life and be there for my family's big moments. My dad's experience was a huge wake-up call, and I decided to change my lifestyle because I love life and want to live it to the fullest. Our hearts are strong, but we still need to take care of them.

How Your Heart Works

For good reason, the heart is often called the engine of the body. Like the engine powering a car, the heart powers your body by pumping blood through a network of highways also known as your blood vessels. The blood delivers essential nutrients and oxygen to every cell, keeping your body running smoothly. The heart's constant, rhythmic pumping provides our organs the vital supplies they need to function. Without this literally life-giving blood, a heart would sputter much like a car that doesn't have a well-maintained engine.

A muscular organ about the size of your fist, your heart sits just behind and slightly left of your breastbone. Your heart has four chambers: two upper chambers called atria and two lower chambers called ventricles. The right side of the heart receives oxygen-poor blood from the body and pumps it to the lungs where it picks up oxygen. The left side receives oxygen-rich blood from the lungs and pumps it throughout the body. This efficient system ensures that every part of the body gets the oxygenated blood it needs to thrive. Keeping your heart healthy and strong will keep you healthy and ready to enjoy life to the fullest.

But our heart doesn't stay healthy automatically.

What Is Heart Disease?

Heart disease refers to a range of conditions affecting the heart and its ability to function effectively. The term refers to, among other disorders, coronary artery disease (which can lead to heart attacks); heart rhythm problems (arrhythmias); and heart defects you're born with (congenital heart defects). Let's look at some of the most common forms of heart disease.

Coronary artery disease (CAD) is the leading cause of death globally and is responsible for 31% of all deaths. This condition develops when the coronary arteries, which supply the heart with oxygen-rich blood, become clogged with plaque. This plaque buildup slows and reduces the blood flow, and that slowdown can cause symptoms like chest pain or lead to a heart attack. Lifestyle factors such as a diet high in saturated fats, lack of physical activity, smoking, and unmanaged stress significantly contribute to the risk. Preventative measures include maintaining a healthy weight, getting regular cardiovascular exercise, and maintaining a diet low in saturated fats and high in fiber. Additionally, managing stress through techniques like meditation or yoga can also reduce the risk of CAD.

A **heart attack** occurs when blood flow to a part of the heart is blocked for long enough that part of the heart muscle is damaged or dies. In the United States, nearly 805,000 people experience a heart attack each year, highlighting the critical need for everyone to be vigilant about their heart health. Risk factors for heart attacks include high blood pressure, high cholesterol, obesity, smoking, and diabetes. Symptoms may not be dramatic. Among the more subtle symptoms are discomfort in the chest, arms, back, neck, or jaw as well as shortness of breath, nausea, or lightheadedness.

If you experience these symptoms, especially if they are persistent or severe, it's crucial to **seek medical attention promptly**. Early intervention can be lifesaving. Even if you're unsure about what you're experiencing, err on the side of caution and get to a healthcare professional with whom you can discuss your symptoms.

If you've been diagnosed with risk factors or have a family history of heart disease, be extra attentive to these symptoms. Treating them as early warning signs and making lifestyle changes, improving your diet, increasing your physical activity, and no longer smoking, can be vital to preventing a heart attack and enhancing your overall heart health.

Affecting approximately 6.2 million adults in the US, **heart failure** occurs when the heart can't maintain the blood flow necessary to meet the body's needs. It can result from a structural or functional cardiac disorder that impairs the ability of the ventricles to fill with blood or move it along. Symptoms include breathlessness, fatigue, and swelling in the legs and abdomen due to fluid accumulation. Management involves a combination of medications such as diuretics to reduce fluid buildup, ACE inhibitors to lower blood pressure, and lifestyle modifications like reduced salt intake. Advanced heart failure may require more invasive treatments such as implantable devices or a heart transplant.

Arrhythmias are disturbances in the heart's rhythm. These irregular heartbeats, whether too fast, too slow, or erratic and can increase the risk of stroke and heart failure. Conditions such as atrial fibrillation, the most common type of arrhythmia, affect millions of people. Symptoms might include palpitations, fainting, and dizziness. Management strategies include medications to control the rate and rhythm of the heart, lifestyle changes to reduce triggers, and, in some cases, surgical interventions like catheter ablation. Regular monitoring and medical checkups are essential for effectively managing arrhythmias and preventing complications.

And then there's the hidden factor of **cholesterol**, which can be a significant risk factor for heart disease. (Cholesterol is a fatty substance in your blood that your body needs to work right, but too much cholesterol can be a bad thing.) Cholesterol affects men and women alike, and recent studies show that about 1 in 10 people under 30 have high cholesterol. In fact, heart disease is one of the leading causes of death among young adults, though it often goes undiagnosed until later.

One day when I was training to be a doctor, I got curious about my own cholesterol levels. I was 25 years old, feeling strong and healthy, and I wasn't worried at all about my health. But when the machine showed my cholesterol levels, I was stunned. The numbers were alarmingly high, comparable to the results of someone in their 70s. I repeated the test several times, and the results were consistent. What a wake-up call for me!

Even if you're young and feeling fine, you may still be at risk. Whatever your age, be proactive about your heart health, monitor your risk factors, and consult with a healthcare professional if you have any concerns. By addressing these issues early on, making healthier lifestyle choices, and staying informed, you can take control of your heart health and potentially prevent future problems.

Those are steps I had to take so that my story wouldn't end with heart disease. My mother who became a marathon runner and a picture of health and vitality after my dad's heart surgery became my rock of hope and inspiration. Watching her lace up her running shoes and hit the pavement day after day, regardless of the weather or her mood, showed me the strength of human will and the impact of consistent, healthy choices. Her dedication to her own health was not just about avoiding disease; it was about living life to its fullest with energy, zest, and joy.

Her example challenged me to look beyond the immediate pleasures of unhealthy habits and consider the long-term benefits of a healthy lifestyle. I wanted to live not in fear of what might happen but with the intention of making the best of my life and its endless opportunities. Moving away from a stance of passive risk to a path of active prevention, I was on my way to better heart health and, ultimately, a better life.

Let's Beat Heart Disease

Reducing your risk of getting heart disease might seem challenging, yet it's entirely achievable. It's empowering to understand that our daily choices. what we eat, how much we move, what we do about our stress level, and what environments we spend time in can significantly influence for good or bad our risk of developing heart disease.

Dietary Changes: Research shows that a healthy diet can help prevent heart disease. Increasing your vegetable and fruit intake can, for instance, lower blood pressure and reduce the risk of heart disease by up to 20%. Moderation and balance are key: it's not about completely eliminating foods but instead creating a diet rich in whole grains, lean proteins, and a variety of vegetables. According to some studies, reducing one's intake of saturated fat and choosing healthier fats, like those from fish, nuts, and avocados, can decrease the risk of heart disease by up to 30%.

Exercise: Regular physical activity can also protect your heart health. The American Heart Association recommends at least 150 minutes of moderate-intensity aerobic activity each week to improve heart health. Yet about 80% of US adults and adolescents do not get enough exercise. Engaging in regular physical activity can reduce the risk of heart disease by up to 35%. Exercise strengthens the heart muscle, improves blood flow, and can help control weight and reduce stress.

If you're new to exercise or returning after a long hiatus, walking each day is a great starting point, but be sure to talk to your doctor before beginning any new routine. Also, while regular activity is key, it's possible to overdo it. To avoid pushing too hard too soon, listen to your body and be mindful of how you're feeling.

Mental Health: The link between mental health and heart disease is profound. Studies suggest that people with depression have a 64% greater risk of developing coronary artery disease. Stress management techniques, such as mindfulness and yoga, have been shown to lower blood pressure and reduce symptoms of heart disease. Creating a lifestyle that includes time for relaxation, hobbies, and social interactions can significantly improve not only your mental health but your heart health as well.

Positive Environments: Having a supportive social network and spending as much time as possible in positive environments can enhance your quality of life and decrease the risk of heart disease. In fact, strong social relationships can reduce the risk of heart disease by about 30%.

Laughter: Did you know that laughter and a positive outlook can improve heart health? Laughter can decrease stress hormones, reduce artery inflammation, and increase HDL, the "good" cholesterol. HDL ("good") cholesterol helps clear excess cholesterol from your arteries, while LDL ("bad") cholesterol can build up and narrow them. So book that comedy show or meet up with your most upbeat, fun friends. Surrounding yourself with people who bring humor and joy is good for your heart in both senses of the word!

Incorporating these changes into your life isn't merely a defense against heart disease; it's also a step toward a fuller, more vibrant life. While genetics and family history play a role in heart health, lifestyle choices wield a powerful influence. By adopting a diet rich in nutrients, regularly participating in physical activity, managing stress, and spending time with positive people in positive environments, we can dramatically shift the trajectory of our health and enhance our lives. The journey toward heart health can be both rewarding and enjoyable.

One more note. Even if you're already taking a medication like statins to manage cholesterol, lifestyle changes can still make a big difference. In fact, adopting healthier habits has in some cases helped reduce the need for medications. Studies have also found that individuals who prioritize exercise, a heart-healthy diet, and stress management can sometimes reverse early signs of heart disease and improve their overall cardiovascular health. It's never too late to take control of your heart health, and even if medications are necessary, self-care can play a powerful role in reducing your dependence on them and improving the long-term outcomes.

Maria's Cardiac Comeback

> Maria, a 52-year-old cashier in a rural town, felt drained daily. She brushed off chest tightness and shortness of breath as work stress. Without insurance, doctors weren't an option. At a church health fair, a nurse found her blood pressure at 150/95, hinting at hypertension. A low-cost clinic prescribed meds, and Maria made tweaks: she swapped fried foods for frozen veggies and beans, walked 30 minutes daily with a church group, and followed YouTube breathing videos. Six months later, her blood pressure was 130/85, and she danced joyfully at her daughter's wedding.

A Healthy Diet: The Foundation for Heart Health

A balanced, heart-healthy diet is essential to maintaining cardiovascular health. A key aspect of eating wisely is matching your calorie intake to your physical activity. Tracking what you eat can help ensure that you're fueling your body properly and not consuming more than your body needs. A good rule of thumb is to focus on nutrient-dense foods those that provide vitamins and minerals without adding excessive calories, such as leafy greens, berries, lean proteins like fish or chicken, whole grains, and legumes. If, for example, you indulge in a higher-calorie meal, plan some extra activity to balance it out.

When it comes to dairy, not all low-fat options are best for heart health. Cutting down on unhealthy fats is important, but some full-fat dairy products, like full-fat Greek yogurt, can actually be better for you than low-fat options that are filled with added sugar. Choose natural, minimally processed dairy products that offer nutrients without unnecessary sugar.

Saturated fats (typically found in red meat, butter, and full-fat dairy products) and trans fats (commonly found in processed foods like cheap baked goods, margarine, and shortening) are known to increase the risk of heart disease. Reducing your intake of these unhealthy fats and replacing them with healthier options, like olive oil or avocado, can make a big difference in the quality of your diet. Additionally, limiting sugary drinks like sodas and energy drinks helps prevent weight gain and diabetes, both of which increase heart disease risk.

Hope for the Future

In recent years, the field of cardiology has seen remarkable advancements that offer new hope and expanded treatment options for those affected by heart disease. These innovations enhance our ability to diagnose heart conditions, to treat those conditions more effectively, and to improve the quality of life for patients dealing with chronic heart issues. Below is a list of some significant breakthroughs in heart healthcare with ideas about how you can start using them today for your own better heart health:

1. Wearable Technology: Devices like smartwatches and fitness trackers can monitor heart rate, detect irregular heartbeats like atrial fibrillation,

and even measure blood oxygen levels. You probably already have this technology on your smartphone or smartwatch, so take advantage of it. Here's what to look for:

- Resting heart rate: A healthy range is typically 60-100 beats per minute (bpm) for adults. If your resting heart rate consistently falls outside this range, consider consulting a doctor.
- Heart rhythm: Irregular heartbeats or skipped beats can be an early sign of heart issues. If you notice irregularities, get it checked out.
- Blood oxygen levels: Aim for a SpO2 level (the percentage of oxygenated hemoglobin in your blood) between 95% and 100%. If levels consistently fall below this, you should consult your healthcare provider. Use your tech daily to monitor these metrics and consider syncing the data with apps that can track trends over time. This information can be invaluable when discussing your health with your doctor.

2. Cholesterol-Lowering Drugs: New classes of drugs like PCSK9 inhibitors are a promising option for patients who struggle to manage their cholesterol levels using traditional and commonly prescribed statins. Nearly 38 million Americans take statins to manage cholesterol. If you're on statins and not seeing the results you want, ask your doctor about alternative treatments like PCSK9 inhibitors that have shown great potential for lowering bad cholesterol and reducing the risk of heart attacks and strokes in high-risk patients.

3. Regenerative Medicine: One of the most exciting developments in cardiology is the use of stem cells and regenerative therapies to repair damaged heart tissue. Research is ongoing, still largely in the research and clinical trial phase, but the hope is that regenerative medicine can help the heart heal itself, potentially treating heart failure and other chronic conditions. If you or a loved one is dealing with heart disease, ask your specialist whether any cutting-edge treatments or trials are available.

4. Artificial Intelligence (AI) in Cardiology: Specialists are using AI and machine learning to predict patient outcomes, personalize treatments, and manage heart disease more effectively. AI algorithms can analyze vast amounts of data from EKGs, wearable devices, and genetic profiles to identify patterns that may predict heart attacks or other cardiac events. While AI-driven treatments are typically accessed

through specialists, the data you collect on your own wearable devices can help doctors provide you with more tailored care. Don't wait until you're under a specialist's care. Start monitoring your health now and share your data with your healthcare provider for more informed decision-making.

Taking charge of your heart health is within your reach and it's one of the most important investments you can make for your long-term well-being. Remember, small, consistent changes today can lead to meaningful benefits tomorrow. To help you on your journey, I've included practical tools on the following pages designed to support and guide you as you build healthier heart habits.

10 Ways to Keep Your Heart Healthy

1. Balance Your Calories Like a Budget

Think of your body spending energy every day. If you eat more energy (calories) than you spend, that extra energy is stored as fat, putting extra strain on your heart. To achieve a balance between energy in and energy out, use a food tracking app or simply check portion sizes. If weight loss is a goal, cut 250 calories a day (just skip a sugary coffee) to lose half a pound per week with relative ease.

2. Fill Your Plate with Heart-Boosting Foods

A colorful plate leads to a healthy heart. Load up on berries, leafy greens, nuts, fish, and legumes while reducing your intake of processed foods. Swap sugary yogurts for full-fat Greek yogurt, trade white bread for whole grains, and make half your plate veggies.

3. Break Up with Trans Fats and Sugary Drinks

Trans fats and added sugars are like poison for your arteries. They increase inflammation, raise cholesterol, and contribute to heart disease. Simple swaps:

- Trade soda for sparkling water with lemon.
- Use olive oil instead of margarine.
- Snack on nuts instead of chips.

4. Cut Back on Red Meat

Red meat raises cholesterol and increases heart disease risk. Try going meatless one day per week (have Meatless Mondays) and have salmon, lentils, or tofu instead. If you eat red meat, limit it to once or twice a week—and choose lean cuts.

5. Quit Smoking

Smoking damages your heart faster than almost anything else. If quitting feels overwhelming, start by delaying your first cigarette by 30 minutes; try nicotine gum or patches; or call a quitline or use an app for support. Your heart starts healing within 20 minutes of that last cigarette.

6. Change Your Alcohol Intake Before It Changes You

Alcohol raises blood pressure and can weaken your heart over time. Try a mocktail with sparkling water, citrus, and herbs to replace your usual drink.

Keep your drinking to a minimum.

7. Get Moving (After All, Your Heart Is a Muscle)

Just 45 minutes of moderate exercise, five days a week, can lower blood pressure, improve circulation, and strengthen your heart.

8. Add Yoga to Reduce Stress and Improve Circulation

Yoga lowers stress hormones and your blood pressure while improving circulation. If you don't love traditional yoga, try a five-minute deep breathing session or simple stretches before bed.

9. Laugh More, Stress Less

Laughter releases nitric oxide that relaxes blood vessels and lowers blood pressure. So schedule joy in your life. Watch a comedy show, call the friend who always makes you laugh, or find humor in small moments.

10. Surround Yourself with Heart-Healthy People

You are twice as likely to stick to healthy habits if your social circle supports them. Find people who motivate you, inspire you, and encourage you.

Your Action Plan for Heart Health

1. Check Your Heart Score

On a scale of 1-10, how healthy do you feel your heart is right now?

- Do you exercise regularly?
- Do you eat mostly whole foods?
- How often do you check your blood pressure?

Write down one thing you can do to improve heart health and start today.

2. The 7-Day Heart Health Challenge

For the next seven days, commit to one of these heart-friendly habits:

- Swap one processed food for a whole food.
- Walk 20-30 minutes every day.
- Try a meatless meal at least once during these seven days.
- Laugh daily: watch something funny or talk to someone who makes you smile.
- Cut back on sugary drinks.

At the end of the week, evaluate how you're feeling.

3. Create a Heart Health Ritual

Pick one daily habit to protect your heart long-term:

- Start checking your blood pressure.
- Make exercise part of your routine.
- Cut back on alcohol or smoking.

Write down your choice. Putting it in writing will improve the chances that you'll approach your choice as if it's a real commitment.

The small changes you make today will protect your heart for decades to come.

CHAPTER 5

VITAL VESSELS:
ENSURING HEALTHY CIRCULATION

Working in the emergency room of Cook County Hospital meant dealing with life-threatening emergencies. I still remember Mrs. B....

In her late fifties, Mrs. B had lived in Chicago for most of her life. Like many in her community, she had limited access to routine healthcare, often leading to delayed treatment and exacerbated health issues. As I spoke with Mrs. B, she recounted her struggles with health and mobility.

"It started with numbness in my toes," she explained. "Then it just got worse, and before I knew it, my foot was gone."

The amputation of her left leg had been a drastic measure to save her life two years prior. Now with her right leg in similar peril, she faced the grim prospect of losing that leg too. The foul smell emanating from it was a telltale sign of the infection that had taken hold due to poor circulation and unchecked diabetes.

The situation was dire, and her case served as a stark picture of the consequences of underserved communities lacking accessible healthcare. For Mrs. B, the nonexistence of early intervention and preventative care had turned a manageable condition into a life-altering crisis. I had seen this kind of scenario all too often: the emergency room was the last resort for people who had fallen through the cracks of the healthcare system. Mrs. B's situation also highlighted the importance of educating people about the signs of poor circulation, managing conditions like diabetes proactively, and advocating for better healthcare resources where few, if any, exist. Lack of access to medical information and care can turn preventable conditions into tragic and even fatal outcomes.

But back to Mrs. B's heartbreaking situation. A significant contributor to the second amputation was poor circulation. What could she have done and what can you do today to help protect yourself and your loved ones from circulation issues? The good news is, you can start taking some simple steps right now to support healthy circulation and avoid the complications that come with poor blood flow. Small changes in your daily habits—whether moving more throughout the day, eating foods that promote healthy blood flow, or staying hydrated—can make a big difference. The earlier you begin to take care of your circulatory health, the more you can reduce the risk of serious issues like blood clots, swelling, and even heart disease. What you can learn in this chapter can have a lasting impact on your health and on the lives of those people you care about.

Why Circulation Matters

Think of your circulatory system as the world's most efficient superhighway with millions of roads and pathways crisscrossing to deliver vital supplies to every corner of your body. This intricate network of veins and arteries, spanning over 60,000 miles, ensures that every cell receives the oxygen and nutrients it needs to thrive while at the same time efficiently removing waste products.

In this vast network, our arteries carry oxygen-rich blood from the heart to, for instance, the muscles and tissues of the legs. These vessels are both strong and elastic, designed to withstand the high pressure of the blood being forcefully pumped by the heart. This oxygenated blood is the lifeblood of our leg muscles, empowering us to walk, run, and jump.

Conversely, veins act as the blood's return pathway. Once the muscles have used the oxygen, depleting it from the blood, the veins carry this now-oxygen-poor blood back to the heart. Unique to veins are their one-way valves ensuring that blood flows in the correct direction, against gravity and back to the heart. This ingenious system guarantees that every part of the leg, from the external layer of skin to the deep muscle tissues, receives a continuous supply of fresh blood, maintaining not just functionality but also the health and even the aesthetic appeal of the legs.

When blood circulates unhindered, legs benefit from a consistent supply of oxygen and nutrients that keeps the skin supple, heals wounds swiftly, and enables muscles to retain their strength and vitality. Conversely, compromised circulation can lead to numerous issues, ranging from varicose veins and swelling to painful ulcers and, in extreme cases, the risk of amputation.

Peripheral artery disease (PAD), a condition where narrowed arteries reduce blood flow to the limbs, affects approximately 8.5 million Americans, according to the American Heart Association. The occurrence of PAD increases with age, affecting up to 20% of individuals over 60. Keeping the circulatory system in optimal condition is crucial for preserving the health and functionality of the legs. Individuals with circulatory issues may experience anxiety and depression due to the chronic nature of their conditions and the resulting limitations on daily activities and lifestyle. People may feel embarrassed about the visible signs of circulatory problems, like varicose veins or skin ulcers, leading to self-consciousness, social withdrawal, isolation, and loneliness. We can avoid all those negatives when we take care of our circulatory system.

When Arteries go Wrong

Just as traffic slows down when highways suffer from congestion due to buildup and blockages, blood slows down when arteries suffer from plaque buildup (atherosclerosis). Plaque, a sticky substance composed of fat, cholesterol, calcium, and other materials found in the blood, can accumulate on the inner walls of arteries. Over time, this buildup narrows the arteries, making it harder for blood to flow through. If some plaque breaks free, a blood clot may result and block the flow of blood entirely. Clearly, the consequences of plaque buildup can be serious and life-threatening, leading to conditions such as coronary artery disease, carotid artery disease, peripheral artery disease, and stroke.

Just as road workers clear debris and fix potholes, we must deal with the plaque buildup that exists and, ideally, manage the factors that contribute to that buildup. To be specific, we need to maintain a diet low in saturated fats and cholesterol; exercise regularly to improve circulation and strengthen the heart; and avoid smoking, which can damage the inner lining of the arteries. By taking control of our health in those three ways, we ensure that our arteries remain open, allowing life-sustaining blood to flow freely to every part of our body.

Leonard Takes the Long Way Home

> Leonard, a 64-year-old retired bus mechanic, had always been on his feet until walking to the mailbox left his calves aching. He started hiding it, pausing mid-walk to "check something" or lean on a fence. At first, he blamed it on age or stiff joints. But when even short walks made his legs burn, he finally saw his doctor.
>
> A vascular ultrasound showed peripheral artery disease his leg arteries were narrowing. Leonard didn't smoke, but years of poor eating, high blood pressure, and long hours sitting had caught up. His doctor prescribed meds and gave him a simple, uncomfortable challenge: walk more, not less.
>
> Leonard started slow. One block. Then two. Even when it burned, he kept moving. He swapped chips for roasted almonds, took blood pressure meds consistently, and added a salad to lunch most days. After 12 weeks, Leonard could walk the entire grocery store without stopping.
>
> He didn't just build stamina, he rebuilt trust in his body. For the first time in years, Leonard stopped taking the shortcut. He took the long way and felt proud doing it.

Veins and Valves

Your veins bring blood back to the heart after they have delivered oxygen and nutrients to the body's tissues. The uniqueness of veins lies in their one-way valves that act as the traffic controllers of the venous system, ensuring that blood flows in one direction toward the heart and against gravity, a real challenge for blood coming from the legs. When these valves fail to work properly, blood can pool in the veins, leading to various complications. According to the Society for Vascular Surgery, about 20 to 25 million Americans have varicose veins, a common condition often resulting from valve failure and underscoring the crucial role of these valves in maintaining proper circulation.

Muscles surrounding the veins also play a crucial role in aiding circulation. During physical activity, these muscles contract and squeeze the veins, helping to push the blood back to the heart. Often referred to as the muscle pump, this essential action is a key reason why regular exercise is critical to circulatory health. In fact, a sedentary lifestyle can significantly increase the risk of circulatory issues. We all need to get up and move around every day. If you work at a desk or spend a lot of time driving, take regular breaks to stretch your legs and get your blood flowing. Even a quick walk or a few minutes of stretching can make a big difference in keeping your circulation healthy.

Maintaining good circulation in the legs is essential for overall health, enabling you to stay active and enjoy a high quality of life. Good leg circulation ensures that waste products are efficiently removed and that nutrients and oxygen are adequately supplied, which is essential for overall vitality and energy. This efficient exchange helps prevent the buildup of toxins in the blood, reducing the risk of conditions like atherosclerosis, a major contributor to cardiovascular disease.

Poor circulation in the legs can force the heart to work harder to pump blood through narrowed or blocked arteries, which can lead to increased blood pressure and eventually heart strain. Over time, this added strain can increase the risk of heart failure or other cardiac complications. You'll find strategies to ensure optimal circulation later on. Some of those complications we'll look at now.

Pain and Cramping

Are you concerned about your leg health? Do you get pain or cramping? Peripheral artery disease (PAD), which typically affects the legs, can be a precursor to more serious cardiovascular issues. It serves as an early warning system for the health of your arteries.

One of the most common symptoms of PAD is claudication, a term referring to pain or cramping in the legs or hips during activities like walking or climbing stairs. This pain typically goes away with rest and returns when the activity resumes. Other symptoms include numbness or weakness in the legs; coldness in the lower leg or foot; sores on the toes, feet, or legs that won't heal; a change in the color of the legs; hair loss or slower hair growth on the feet and legs; and slower growth of toenails. If you are concerned about any of these symptoms, talk to your doctor.

Several factors increase the risk of developing PAD, including smoking, diabetes, high blood pressure, high cholesterol, obesity, and a sedentary lifestyle. Age is also a significant factor, with the risk increasing for people over 50. Family history of cardiovascular disease can also elevate the risk of PAD. People with a history of heart disease, stroke, or other vascular diseases are more likely to develop PAD.

Deep Vein Thrombosis

Deep vein thrombosis (DVT) is a serious condition that occurs when a blood clot forms in a deep vein, typically in the lower leg, thigh, or pelvis. These clots can obstruct blood flow, causing swelling and pain in the affected area. If a clot breaks loose, it can travel through the bloodstream to the lungs, resulting in a potentially life-threatening condition known as a pulmonary embolism.

Among the most common symptoms of DVT are swelling in one leg; leg pain or tenderness that may feel like a cramp; reddish or bluish skin discoloration; and a feeling of warmth in the affected leg. Early detection of DVT is crucial to preventing complications.

The following factors increase the risk of developing DVT:

- Extended periods of immobility, such as long car or plane trips when the legs remain still for long periods and blood flow slows
- Certain medical conditions, such as cancer, heart disease, and inflammatory bowel disease, as well as a personal or family history of DVT or pulmonary embolism
- Major surgery and significant injuries, particularly involving the legs or abdomen, that cause prolonged immobility and damage to blood vessels
- Smoking, obesity, and a sedentary lifestyle that contribute to poor circulation and the likelihood of clot formation

- Pregnancy, hormone replacement therapy, and birth control pills that change hormone levels and can contribute to blood clotting

Several preventative measures are essential to reducing the risk of DVT. Regular physical activity is crucial for maintaining healthy blood flow, with exercises like walking, leg lifts, and calf raises especially during long periods of immobility. Wearing compression stockings can prevent blood from pooling in the leg veins and reduce the risk of clot formation. Staying well-hydrated is crucial because dehydration can lead to thicker blood, increasing the risk of clotting.

During long trips, make a point of periodically standing up, stretching, and moving around. If even that isn't possible, flexing and extending the ankles frequently can encourage blood flow. Maintaining a healthy weight, not smoking, and managing chronic conditions like diabetes and hypertension are also important preventative measures.

How to Have Good Circulation

- **Stay Active:** Regular physical activity promotes blood flow and strengthens the muscles that support your veins. Walking, cycling, and swimming are great choices. Aim for at least 30 minutes of moderate exercise on most days of the week to keep your circulation strong.
- **Elevate Your Legs:** Elevating your legs above your heart for 15-20 minutes a day can help improve circulation and reduce swelling. A simple way to do this is to lie on your back with a pillow under your feet. Gravity will help the blood flow back to your heart.
- **Compression Stockings:** Wearing compression stockings can prevent blood from pooling in your leg veins and improve blood flow back to your heart. These socks are especially helpful after surgery, on long plane flights, and if your job requires you to stand for long periods.
- **Hydrate Well:** Drinking enough water is crucial for maintaining the volume of blood in your body and keeping circulation smooth. Light yellow urine indicates you're staying properly hydrated.
- **Maintain a Healthy Weight:** Excess weight that puts extra pressure on your veins can impede blood flow. Maintaining a healthy weight helps reduce this pressure and keeps circulation optimal.

- **Supportive Network:** Surround yourself with people who support your health goals. A good support system encourages you to stay active, eat well, and maintain positive lifestyle habits. With that support, you'll have an easier time sticking to your health objectives.

- **Stretch Regularly:** Stretching exercises, especially those targeting the legs, can enhance circulation and flexibility, thereby reducing the risk of circulatory problems.

- **Healthy Diet:** A diet rich in vegetables, whole grains, and lean proteins can help reduce inflammation and plaque buildup in arteries. Foods high in antioxidants, such as berries, nuts, and green leafy vegetables, are particularly beneficial for blood vessel health.

- **Avoid Smoking:** Giving up tobacco can significantly improve circulation and reduce your risk of vascular diseases.

- **Limit Alcohol Consumption:** Drink alcohol in moderation; excessive alcohol intake can lead to health issues that affect circulation.

- **Regular Checkups:** Regular visits to your healthcare provider can help with the detection and management of conditions like diabetes, high blood pressure, and high cholesterol that may affect circulation.

- **Footwear Choices**: Wearing comfortable, supportive shoes is key to good circulation and reducing the risk of foot and leg problems. If you spend long hours standing or walking, choose shoes that have good arch support and adequate cushioning. You also need a proper fit to avoid putting pressure on your veins. If you're not sure what's best for your feet, consult a podiatrist who can recommend shoes or insoles tailored to your needs and able to help prevent circulatory issues.

- **Monitor Your Leg Health:** Pay attention to any signs of poor circulation, such as persistent swelling, changes in skin color, or increased leg fatigue. Don't hesitate to seek medical advice if you have any concerns.

Cold and Heat Therapy

Did you know that cold and heat therapy can improve circulation? **Cold therapy** helps reduce swelling and inflammation, and **heat therapy** increases blood flow to specific areas. You can try these methods at home to support your circulatory health:

- **Cold Therapy**: Cold showers, cold-water swimming, or using an ice pack on sore muscles can all help reduce inflammation and encourage blood to flow more efficiently after the source of the cold is removed. Cold-water swimming in particular has been shown to stimulate circulation as the body works to warm itself back up. A cold shower or a quick dip in cool water can also help boost circulation.
- **Heat Therapy**: Applying a heating pad, taking a warm bath, or using a warm compress can help dilate blood vessels and improve blood flow to an area. Heat therapy is especially effective for increasing circulation in stiff muscles and joints. Using heat after cold therapy can further enhance circulation as the veins and arteries move from a constricted to a dilated state.

These simple techniques can be done at home to promote better blood flow and alleviate circulatory discomfort.

Foods and Supplements for Good Circulation

What you eat plays a big role in supporting healthy circulation. Certain foods and supplements can improve blood flow, strengthen blood vessels, and reduce inflammation. Always look to whole foods before turning to supplements, but both can help promote better circulation. Here are some key options to consider for improving circulation:

- Citrus fruits including oranges, lemons, and grapefruits that are rich in Vitamin C strengthen capillary walls.
- Beets are high in nitrates that widen blood vessels.
- Omega-3 fatty acids in oily fish like salmon, mackerel, and sardines have omega-3s that reduce inflammation. Vegans and vegetarians can consider algae-based supplements that offer a plant-based source of omega-3s.
- L-Arginine helps produce nitric oxide that relaxes blood vessels.
- Magnesium dilates blood vessels and lowers blood pressure. Foods rich in magnesium include bananas, spinach, and almonds.
- Coenzyme Q10 (CoQ10) supports heart health and circulation by improving symptoms of heart failure and reducing blood pressure.

- Ginkgo biloba boosts circulation especially in the legs and also enhances cognitive function.
- Vitamin E acts like a blood thinner and antioxidant. You can find Vitamin E in foods like sunflower seeds, almonds, and spinach.
- Garlic extract supports blood pressure regulation and improves arterial health.
- Flavonoids, found in cocoa and green tea, improve blood vessel function. Drink green tea or enjoy a small piece of dark chocolate with high cocoa content to get your daily dose of these circulation-boosting compounds.
- Capsaicin, present in spicy foods like chili peppers, increases blood flow when applied as a cream or consumed as a supplement.

Foods to Avoid

Just as certain foods can improve circulation, others can harm it. Limiting the following foods can help protect your blood vessels and improve your overall heart health:

- **High-Sodium Foods:** Too much salt can lead to high blood pressure, damaging your blood vessels and reducing circulation. The recommended limit is no more than 2,300 mg of sodium per day, but aiming for less than 1,500 mg is even better. Reduce the salt in your diet by cooking at home, choosing low-sodium options, and cutting back on processed and packaged foods.
- **Trans and Saturated Fats:** Found in foods like fried snacks, processed meats, and baked goods, these fats contribute to plaque buildup in your arteries, restricting blood flow and increasing the risk of heart disease.
- **Processed Foods:** Often high in sodium, added sugars, and unhealthy fats, processed foods can negatively affect circulation. Choose instead whole, minimally processed foods.

Adopting these strategies and making other informed lifestyle choices can significantly improve circulation in your legs, leading to healthier, more vibrant legs and greater well-being overall.

Maintain Stable Blood Sugar

Switching now to the topic of sugar, know that keeping your blood sugar levels within a healthy range is essential for good circulation and overall cardiovascular health. Blood sugar levels that are too high or that fluctuate frequently can damage the blood vessels and nerves that control circulation, especially in the legs and feet. Individuals with diabetes or those at risk of developing it should be especially aware of their blood sugar.

Why Stable Blood Sugar Matters

A consistently high level of blood sugar can lead to the hardening and narrowing of blood vessels, a condition known as atherosclerosis. Over time, this condition restricts blood flow to various parts of the body, especially the extremities, making it harder for oxygen and nutrients to reach cells. Poor blood circulation in the legs and feet increases the risk of complications like peripheral artery disease (PAD), slower healing, and even the development of ulcers. Individuals with diabetes face an increased risk of nerve damage (neuropathy), which can further affect circulation and lead to more serious complications, including the risk of amputation.

Balanced Meals for Stable Blood Sugar

Maintaining stable blood sugar levels starts with eating balanced meals that include a healthy mix of fiber, protein, and healthy fats. Here's how each plays a role:

- **Fiber:** Whole grains, fruits, vegetables, and legumes that are rich in fiber help slow down the absorption of sugar into the bloodstream. This prevents sharp spikes in blood sugar after meals, which is important because frequent spikes and crashes can lead to energy swings, increased hunger, and over time, a higher risk of developing insulin resistance or type 2 diabetes. Including fiber-rich foods like lentils, beans, oats, and leafy greens in your diet will support a stable level of blood sugar, helping you feel fuller longer and keeping your energy steady throughout the day.

- **Protein:** In addition to helping keep you full longer than other foods do, protein slows the digestion of carbohydrates, preventing rapid increases in blood sugar. Incorporate into your meals lean proteins like chicken, fish, and tofu or plant-based proteins like chickpeas and quinoa.

- **Healthy Fats:** Healthy fats, such as those found in avocados, olive oil, and nuts, are essential for stabilizing blood sugar. These fats provide energy and help improve insulin sensitivity, which is key to managing blood sugar levels.

Practical Tips for Managing Blood Sugar

- **Portion Control:** Eating smaller, balanced meals at regular intervals throughout the day can help keep the level of blood sugar steady. Large meals, especially those high in refined carbohydrates, can cause spikes in blood sugar. Try eating smaller portions every 3 to 4 hours to avoid drastic fluctuations.

- **Limit Processed Carbohydrates:** Foods like white bread, pastries, and sugary snacks that are quickly digested can cause rapid increases in blood sugar. Swapping these out for whole grains, sweet potatoes, and fiber-rich foods helps prevent sharp rises in glucose levels.

- **Stay Hydrated:** Drinking plenty of water helps keep blood sugar stable by supporting kidney function, which helps remove excess sugar from the bloodstream.

- **Monitor Blood Sugar:** It's crucial that people with diabetes or at risk of diabetes regularly check their blood sugar level; use a blood glucose monitor to track patterns; and discuss any irregularities with their healthcare provider.

- With a focus on eating balanced meals and maintaining stable blood sugar levels, you can significantly improve circulation, reduce the risk of complications, and support long-term heart health.

10 Ways to Help Your Blood Flow

1. Get Moving

Your legs rely on good circulation to stay healthy. Walking, swimming, or cycling for just 30 minutes a day helps pump blood back to your heart, reducing your risk of varicose veins, swelling, and leg fatigue. If you sit for long periods, set a timer so you stand up and move every 30 to 60 minutes.

2. Find a Fitness Tribe

Staying active is easier when you enjoy the process, and having a tribe adds to the enjoyment. Find a walking group, join a cycling class, or take a weekly hike with friends. Working out with people provides a degree of accountability, and this accountability increases consistency and helps healthy habits stick.

3. Cut Out Foods That Clog Your Arteries

Plaque buildup in your arteries blocks blood flow to your legs, leading to pain, numbness, and even serious conditions like peripheral artery disease (PAD). Limiting fried foods, processed meats, and sugary or ultra-processed snacks will help minimize plaque. Instead eat heart-healthy fats, lean proteins, and whole foods. You'll be keeping your circulation strong.

4. Eat More Plant-Based Power

Legumes like chickpeas, lentils, and beans are packed with fiber, protein, and nutrients that boost circulation and improve heart health. Try swapping meat for a plant-based meal once or twice a week to give your blood vessels a break.

5. Take Control of Your Blood Pressure

Check your numbers regularly. An ideal blood pressure is 120/80 mmHg or lower. High blood pressure damages blood vessels and reduces circulation to your legs. If your blood pressure is high, try reducing salt intake, exercising daily, and eating potassium-rich foods like bananas and spinach.

- **Supercharge Your Diet with Cholesterol-Lowering Foods**
- Clear your arteries by adding foods that naturally reduce bad cholesterol (LDL):
- Avocados are rich in heart-healthy fats.
- Almonds and walnuts boost good cholesterol (HDL).
- Dark chocolate (70% or higher) improves circulation.

- Garlic lowers blood pressure and fights plaque buildup.

7. Keep Blood Sugar Steady

An unstable level of blood sugar damages blood vessels, leading to poor circulation, swelling, and nerve pain in the legs. To keep levels steady:

- Eat fiber-rich foods like oats, beans, and berries.
- Pair carbohydrates with protein and healthy fats to slow sugar spikes.
- Avoid sugary drinks and refined carbs.

8. Quit Smoking (Your Legs Will Thank You!)

Smoking damages arteries, weakens circulation, and increases the risk of blood clots. The good news? Within 20 minutes after you smoke your last cigarette, your blood pressure improves, and within a few weeks, circulation starts to recover. If quitting feels overwhelming, start by cutting back or switching to nicotine alternatives.

9. Boost Your Nutrients for Stronger Legs

Your legs need B vitamins, Vitamin D, and magnesium to support circulation, nerve function, and muscle strength. If you get leg cramps, fatigue, or tingling, check your nutrient intake.

- Vitamin D – salmon, fortified dairy, and exposure to sunlight
- B vitamins – whole grains, eggs, and leafy greens
- Magnesium – nuts, seeds, and bananas

10. Add Power-Packed Seeds to Your Diet

Packed with omega-3s, fiber, and anti-inflammatory properties, flaxseeds and chia seeds are circulation superheroes. Here are three ways to add them to your diet:

- Sprinkle flaxseed on oatmeal or yogurt.
- Add chia seeds to smoothies.
- Mix these seeds into salads for a nutrient boost.

You'll notice there's no formal action plan at the end of this chapter—and that's on purpose. Taking care of your vital vessels, from your heart to your brain to every blood vessel in between is essential. It's understanding the principles that protect your circulation and putting them into practice in a way that fits your life.

CHAPTER 6

BREAKING FREE OF UNHEALTHY HABITS:

YOU CAN BE A HEALTHIER YOU

L iam excelled in school, and his academic abilities earned him numerous awards and scholarships. He struggled, however, with social interactions and began using alcohol to cope with the stress. Liam went on to attend a top university and continued to excel academically. His drinking habit worsened, and he often found himself attending late-night parties and missing classes.

After graduating with honors, Liam secured a prestigious position at a research institute. He met and married a woman who admired his intelligence and ambition, but as his addiction intensified, the cracks in their relationship began to show. Financially, his family suffered as Liam wasted money on alcohol and short-lived pleasures.

Fearing he might lose everything, Liam sought help. He went to rehab, attended meetings, and got professional support. He was making progress and starting to put the pieces of his life back together. Just as Liam seemed on the verge of a lasting recovery, tragedy struck: he died from a brain aneurysm. His family was left grappling with their grief, mourning both Liam and the years all of them had lost to his addiction.

As Liam's story highlights, people struggling with addiction need strong support systems. As a doctor, I meet many patients who drink too much alcohol, are hooked on drugs, are addicted to porn, or wrestle with habits that seemed so harmless at first but have had a significant negative impact on their health and well-being. Liam's tragic story reminds us that addiction and harmful habits don't merely affect an individual; those addictions affect families and relationships. Many unhealthy habits, some easier to hide than others, can gradually take a toll.

In this chapter, we'll take a closer look at the common and less-than-healthy habits of drinking, smoking, overeating, and spending too much time on screens; why we might fall into them; and how they can make life tougher for us physically, mentally, and emotionally. We'll consider why that extra soda isn't really our friend, how sitting around all day can be as bad for our health as eating junk food, and why it's sometimes so hard to put down our phones. Most important, we'll talk about how to break free from these unhealthy behaviors. No matter how long these habits have been part of your life, you can make a change. Every day offers you a new chance to improve your health, your well-being, and your future.

How Unhealthy Habits Affect Us

We all have habits, some good and some not so good. The not-so-good ones like drinking too much soda, spending all day on the couch, using our phones too much can really mess with our health and happiness.

Maybe you know someone who smokes or who spends every free minute on the phone, barely looking up. Or maybe you've noticed how you feel after sitting around all day versus going out and being active. These behaviors might seem OK or even fun at first, but they can have some serious downsides: we may find ourselves getting sick more often, being tired all the time, or feeling sad or stressed out. At some point these patterns can become unhealthy habits.

The cool part is, we're going to talk about how to beat these habits. The key is not willpower: it's not clenching your teeth as you try desperately not to eat the cookie that's right in front of you. The key is understanding why we do these things and then figuring out smart ways to change, like swapping that soda for water or making sure we move around more instead of sitting all day. Small changes we can make add up to big results.

Managing these unhealthy habits is super-important because we'll then feel better, do more stuff we love, and be happier and healthier overall. It's like leveling up in real life. Granted, making these changes might seem hard at first, but every single one of us has the power to change our habits and make better choices. Sometimes we might need a little help from friends, family, or doctors, and that's OK. That first step will be the hardest.

Why We Like Habits That Aren't Good for Us

Whether they involve substances like alcohol and nicotine or behaviors like excessive screen time or eating, unhealthy habits often share neurological pathways with those involving the brain's reward system. This system is regulated by neurotransmitters, the chemicals in the brain that transmit messages between neurons and regulate that reward system. Maybe you'll recognize the names of some of them:

1. **Dopamine:** Often referred to as the "feel good" neurotransmitter, dopamine is released during pleasurable situations. As it stimulates you to seek out the pleasurable activity or substance again, this neurotransmitter reinforces and regulates behaviors and emotions. Virtually all types of addictions—whether it's drugs, a fulfilling meal, or winning a video game—involve the dopamine pathway.
2. **Serotonin:** This neurotransmitter contributes to feelings of well-being and happiness. Various behaviors and substances that influence mood, anxiety, and happiness affect the level of serotonin. Low levels are often associated with depression that might drive individuals to engage in certain unhealthy habits as a way to self-medicate and temporarily boost their serotonin level.
3. **Norepinephrine (Noradrenaline):** Associated with arousal and alertness, norepinephrine plays a role in our response to stress, heightening the effects of stimulant use or risky behaviors. Norepinephrine can make these experiences feel more thrilling and lead to dependence on them as the individual continually tries to recreate that thrill.

4. **GABA (gamma-aminobutyric acid):** GABA is an inhibitory neurotransmitter that helps to dampen neural activity. Substances like alcohol increase GABA's effect, leading to decreased anxiety and a degree of sedation but also impairing cognitive and motor functions. Over time, as the brain becomes accustomed to this heightened GABA activity, it may naturally produce less GABA, leading to a tolerance of that lower level. As a result of their brain producing less GABA, people may need to consume more alcohol or similar substances to achieve the same calming effect, potentially leading to dependence as they seek to feel better.
5. **Endorphins:** These are the body's natural painkillers that also enhance feelings of pleasure. Activities like eating, exercise, and sex can increase endorphins. People seeking to achieve feelings of euphoria or pain relief may become over-reliant on unhealthy habits that spike endorphin levels, particularly those activities involving physical sensations or substances.

The Impact on Your Body

As a doctor, I often witness the devastating effects of alcohol and substance abuse on the body and the mind. The impact of unhealthy habits varies depending on the behavior and the substance involved, but the results generally include the following:

- **Addiction and Dependency:** The repeated use of substances and engagement in certain behaviors can lead to both physical and psychological addiction. The brain becomes accustomed to dopamine surges and begins to rely on the substance or behavior to stimulate pleasure and satisfaction. A cycle of dependency results.
- **Deteriorating Health:** Prolonged engagement in unhealthy habits can lead to severe health problems. Smoking leads to the destruction of lung tissue, lung cancer, and heart disease; excessive alcohol use can cause liver disease and neurological complications; and overeating can result in obesity and metabolic syndrome, a cluster of conditions that increase the risk of heart disease, stroke, and diabetes.
- **Cognitive Decline:** Many substances and behaviors negatively impact cognitive function over time. Prolonged substance abuse, for example,

can impair memory, compromise decision-making abilities, and even reduce brain size.
- **Emotional Instability**: The roller coaster of highs and lows associated with many unhealthy habits can lead to depression, anxiety, or other mood disorders. Frequent dopamine and serotonin fluctuations change the brain's chemistry and destabilize mood regulation.

ALCOHOL

Alcohol seems to be a big part of almost every celebration and get-together, making it feel like a normal, even necessary, part of being social. From clinking glasses in a wedding toast to kicking back with a beer at a BBQ, alcohol is often at the center of the fun. But not often talked about is how alcohol, despite being so common, can cause serious trouble not only for the person drinking it but for their family, their friends, and even people they don't know. Think about the victim of a drunk driver someone simply driving home from work or picking up their kids whose life is forever changed by another person's decision to drink and get behind the wheel. The ripple effects of alcohol misuse can reach far beyond the person holding the drink.

Think of alcohol as that friend who's a lot of fun at first but then starts causing problems as the night goes on. Having a drink now and then isn't a big deal for most people (it's a lot of fun at first), but as the night goes on, when "now and then" turns into "every day", problems arise. Among some of the serious health issues that can result are damage to your liver and your heart. Alcohol can also change how people act, making them say or do things they wouldn't usually and sometimes hurting others or themselves by making unsafe choices.

Despite that reality, ads, movies, and TV shows often show drinking as something cool or glamorous and absolutely free of any downside. Young people especially can conclude that drinking is a good way to fit in with a group or deal with stress. They're either ignoring or are oblivious to the real risks of alcohol.

Because alcohol is so widely accepted and even expected in so many places, we can easily forget that alcohol is a really strong substance that can have major negative effects on our bodies and minds. That's why having the full picture is critical to making choices that are healthy and safe for both the short- and the long-term.

- According to the World Health Organization, every year alcohol results in 3 million deaths globally, accounting for 5.3% of all deaths.
- Alcohol is the leading risk factor for premature mortality and disability among those aged 15 to 49 years, and it is responsible for 10% of all deaths in this age group.
- The risk of developing breast cancer increases by 7% to 10% for each 10 grams of alcohol women consume daily. To put this statistic into perspective, a standard glass of wine (about 5 oz) contains approximately 14 grams of alcohol, and a single shot of spirits (1.5 oz) contains roughly 14 grams as well. A single small glass of wine per day can increase a woman's breast cancer risk.

How Alcohol Causes Liver Damage

When you drink alcohol, it gets into your bloodstream and travels into cells all around your body. Inside the cells, alcohol creates harmful substances called free radicals, and these little troublemakers cause chaos. They damage important parts of the cell, including proteins, fats, and even the DNA that serves as the cell's instruction manual.

Your cells do have a cleanup crew called antioxidants that try to get rid of these troublemakers. But if there's too much alcohol and therefore too many free radicals, the cleanup crew can't keep up. It's like having a small team of cleaners trying to clean up the entire city after a massive storm. They just can't handle it.

Sometimes the damage from alcohol is too much for a cell to handle, and it can't be fixed. When this happens, the cell goes through a process called programmed cell death, or apoptosis. This process is a bit like a self-destruct mechanism built into cells that prevents them from turning into cancer cells or causing other problems. Although apoptosis is a normal part of keeping your body healthy, too much cell death, especially in important organs like the liver, can lead to serious health issues.

The liver gets hit especially hard by alcohol. It's like the storm's main target. The liver processes the alcohol, but that task can lead to liver cells dying. Over time, as more and more liver cells die, the result can be liver diseases like fatty liver, hepatitis, and eventually cirrhosis, where the liver is so scarred that it can't do its job properly.

Back to our storm analogy, drinking too much alcohol is like throwing a huge, wild party in your body. When the storm causes a lot of damage, sometimes the city's workers (your cells) can't clean up fast enough, leading to parts of the city (like your liver) getting really damaged. Again, that's why it's critical to think about how much alcohol you're drinking and how often. To keep everything running smoothly, you have to give your body a chance to recover.

To help you stay in control and to protect your health, know the recommended limits for alcohol consumption. For most adults, health guidelines suggest no more than 14 units of alcohol per week, spread over several days, with at least two alcohol-free days. A unit is roughly equivalent to a small glass of wine (125ml) or a single shot of spirits (25ml). Regularly exceeding these limits can increase your risk of long-term health issues.

If you feel you're struggling to cut back on drinking or need support, see read further for advice on how to seek help.

Now let's look at the impact of alcohol on various parts of the body:

Your Central Nervous System: Alcohol's effects on the brain are immediate and often quickly evident in a person's change of mood, cognition, and behavior. As it disrupts the balance of neurotransmitters, which are the brain's chemical messengers, alcohol leads to the initial feelings of euphoria associated with drinking. However, as consumption continues, alcohol impairs judgment, coordination, and reaction times, contributing to risky behaviors and accidents. Long-term excessive drinking can lead to persistent changes in brain function and structure, contributing to memory loss, cognitive decline, and an increased risk of mental health disorders.

Cardiovascular Effects: Although moderate alcohol consumption has been linked to certain cardiovascular benefits such as a possible increase in HDL ("good") cholesterol or reduced risk of coronary artery disease in some studies these benefits are often overstated and depend heavily on individual factors like genetics, lifestyle, and overall health. Excessive drinking, on the other hand, can have harmful effects. It can cause cardiomyopathy, a condition where the heart muscle weakens and becomes unable to pump blood effectively. Alcohol also contributes to hypertension (high blood pressure), irregular heart rhythms (arrhythmias), and an increased risk of stroke

Cancer Risk: A known carcinogen, cancer is particularly associated with cancers of the mouth, throat, esophagus, liver, breast, and colon. The risk of cancer increases with the amount of alcohol consumed. Alcohol contributes to cancer, for instance, with the production of acetaldehyde, which can damage DNA and proteins, and the increased levels of certain hormones (like estrogen) associated with cancer risk.

Digestive System: Alcohol can irritate the gastrointestinal tract, leading to inflammation of the stomach lining (gastritis) and the pancreas (pancreatitis). These conditions can be painful and, if they're not managed, may lead to serious complications. Chronic alcohol use can also interfere with the absorption of nutrients, leading to deficiencies that impact overall health.

Immune System: Excessive alcohol consumption weakens the immune system, making the body more susceptible to infections. Because alcohol can impair the body's ability to fight off pathogens, it has been linked to an increased risk of pneumonia and tuberculosis. This compromised immune response can also affect the body's ability to recover from injuries and infections.

Alcohol and Sleep

Initially, alcohol might seem like a good sleep aid because it can make you feel drowsy and help you fall asleep. Alcohol has this effect because it's a depressant: it can slow down your brain and body, making you feel more relaxed.

But the impact of alcohol changes as the night goes on. Even though alcohol might help you doze off faster, it messes with the quality of your sleep. Here's how:

- **Sleep Cycles:** Your sleep has different stages, from light sleep to deep sleep and then dreamy REM (Rapid Eye Movement) sleep. Alcohol can shorten the REM stage, which is important for memory and learning. So even if you're sleeping, you're not getting the restorative rest your body and brain need.

- **Waking Up:** As the alcohol wears off, your body shifts back into lighter sleep stages, making you more likely to wake up in the middle of the night. That's why you might find yourself staring at the ceiling at 3 a.m. even though you fell asleep easily.

- **Snoring and Breathing:** Alcohol relaxes the muscles in your throat, making you snore more and even leading to breathing problems like sleep apnea while you sleep.

- **Melatonin Production:** Alcohol can mess with the production of melatonin, the hormone that helps regulate your sleep-wake cycle. This reduced melatonin level can make it harder for your body to stick to its natural rhythm.

- **Timing Is Everything:** Drinking alcohol close to bedtime can shift the timing of your internal clock, making it harder to fall asleep at your usual time.

- **Light and Dark Cues:** Your circadian rhythm, your internal 24-hour clock, relies on light and dark cues to function correctly. Since alcohol disrupts sleep quality and patterns, it indirectly messes with these cues, further throwing off your body's internal clock.

At the end of the day, alcohol is one of those things that can feel harmless even routine until it's not. The key is being intentional: knowing your limits, understanding the risks, and recognizing that sometimes the healthiest choice is simply saying no. Alcohol may be common in celebrations, but protecting your health is worth raising a different kind of glass – to a clear mind and strong heart.

SMOKING

When you smoke cigarettes or use tobacco products, you're inhaling nicotine along with about 7,000 other chemicals, many of which are toxic. Within seconds of your taking a puff, nicotine reaches your brain, stimulates the release of adrenaline and dopamine, and results in temporary feelings of pleasure and energy. Nicotine also raises your heart rate and blood pressure, putting a strain on your heart.

In fact, smoking is notorious for damaging nearly every organ in your body. It's a leading cause of cancer, not just in parts of the body directly exposed like the lungs, mouth, and throat, but also in organs like the bladder and pancreas that you wouldn't immediately connect with smoking. Smoking also raises the risk of heart disease, stroke, lung diseases, and type 2 diabetes. The impact on lung health is particularly severe, leading to conditions like chronic obstructive pulmonary disease (COPD) and emphysema.

According to the World Health Organization, tobacco kills more than 8 million people worldwide each year. More than 7 million of those deaths are the result of direct tobacco use, while around 1.2 million are the result of nonsmokers being exposed to secondhand smoke. Also, the Centers for Disease Control and Prevention (CDC) reports that smoking increases the risk of dying from all causes, not just those linked to tobacco use. The life expectancy for smokers is at least 10 years shorter than that of nonsmokers.

Smoking also impacts your immune system. Tobacco puts your body's defense system under constant attack, making it harder for you to fight off infections. That's why smokers often get sick more easily and take longer to recover from illnesses.

The Impact on Appearance

Ever wonder why smokers sometimes look older than they are? The chemicals in cigarettes can speed up the aging process of your skin, leading to wrinkles and a dull complexion. The more than 7,000 chemicals in cigarette smoke reduce blood flow, deprive the skin of oxygen and essential nutrients, and lead to premature aging, making smokers look older than their nonsmoking peers. Smoking can also reduce the production of collagen and elastin, proteins that keep skin firm and elastic, thereby accelerating the formation of wrinkles and fine lines particularly around the eyes and mouth. In addition to causing significantly more wrinkles and sagging skin than nonsmokers deal with, smoking can also mean a sallow, uneven complexion. As the toxins in cigarette smoke cause blood vessels to constrict, the reduced blood flow leads to a pale or grayish skin tone.

Additionally, the tar and nicotine in tobacco can leave hard-to-remove stains on the skin and a yellowish-brown residue on your teeth. Besides being unattractive, that residue on the teeth can contribute to tooth decay and gum disease. Smokers are twice as likely as nonsmokers to develop gum disease and therefore more likely to lose teeth and require dental treatment.

The effects of smoking on appearance are not limited to the skin and mouth. Smoking can also cause hair to become brittle and dry, leading to increased hair loss. The toxins in cigarette smoke can damage hair follicles, impairing growth and leading to thinning hair. Smokers are more likely to experience premature graying and hair loss than nonsmokers.

Finally, smoking contributes to bad breath, often referred to as "smoker's breath." The lingering odor of tobacco smoke in the mouth and lungs can be unpleasant and persistent. This odor is due to the accumulation of smoke particles in the oral cavity, which can also lead to dry mouth, further exacerbating bad breath. Unsurprisingly, smokers are more likely to suffer from chronic halitosis than nonsmokers.

Quitting smoking is one of the most powerful decisions you can make for your health no matter your age, your history, or how long you've been smoking, it's never too late to stop and start healing.

Corey Ditches the Vape

> Corey, a 17-year-old high school junior, started vaping in the locker room after soccer practice. It felt harmless and everyone did it. But soon, he was hitting his vape before class, after school, and even in the bathroom between periods. He told himself it was just stress.
>
> When he started waking up wheezing and couldn't finish a full game without coughing, his coach pulled him aside. That moment hit hard. With support from his mom and a school counselor, Marcus made a plan: delete the vape delivery apps, tell his friends, and set a quit date.
>
> He chewed gum during cravings, did push-ups when stressed, and logged his progress in a notes app. His coach texted him daily to check in. Six weeks later, Marcus was breathing easier and back to full games and no vape in sight.

Vaping

Often perceived as a safer alternative to smoking, vaping involves inhaling aerosolized liquids (e-liquids) containing nicotine, flavorings, and other substances. While it eliminates some of the combustible toxins found in cigarette smoke, vaping introduces its own set of health risks.

The inhalation of nicotine and chemicals like propylene glycol and glycerin can irritate and damage lung tissue. The aerosols inhaled during vaping contain fine particles that can be deeply inhaled into the lungs, causing inflammation and potential damage to lung tissue. Research published in the American Journal of Preventative Medicine found that vaping is associated with a 34% increased risk of chronic lung diseases, including asthma and chronic bronchitis. The inhalation of other additives in e-liquids has been linked to health issues. Some chemicals used for flavoring, such as diacetyl, are associated with serious lung disease, including bronchiolitis obliterans, commonly known as "popcorn lung." Finally, vaping is at the root of a condition known as EVALI (e-cigarette or vaping product use-associated lung injury). According to statistics from the Centers for Disease Control and Prevention (CDC), 2,807 cases of EVALI and 68 deaths were attributed to vaping-related lung injuries in the United States in 2019. In that same year, over 27% of middle- and high-school students in the US reported using e-cigarettes, making it a significant public health concern.

The long-term effects of vaping are still unknown, raising concerns about its safety. The Food and Drug Administration (FDA) continues to investigate the health impacts of e-cigarettes. According to the 2020 National Youth Tobacco Survey, over 3.6 million youth in the US use e-cigarettes, making the potential for widespread health issues significant. More and more, public health initiatives focus on reducing vaping among young people to prevent the onset of nicotine addiction and related health concerns.

The Impact on Your Body

We return to smoking and the continuing list of its negative impact:

Reproduction: Men who smoke may find themselves dealing with reduced sperm quality and, because smoking affects blood flow necessary for an erection, impotence. Women who smoke face increased risks of infertility, complications during pregnancy, and delivering babies with low birth weight. Also, nicotine and other toxins found in cigarettes can cross the placenta, affecting fetal development.

Digestion: Nicotine and other chemicals in cigarettes disrupt the normal function of the digestive system, leading to discomfort and a higher risk of developing such gastrointestinal diseases as ulcers and cancer of the digestive tract. Smoking can also exacerbate inflammatory conditions like Crohn's disease and contribute to a higher risk of serious health issues.

Bones: Smoking affects the body's ability to absorb calcium, which is crucial for strong bones, so smokers are at greater risk for bone fractures and osteoporosis. Over time, reduced bone density can also contribute to a slower healing time when a bone does break.

Nicotine Addiction: The addictive nature of nicotine makes smoking and vaping hard to stop. Nicotine stimulates the release of dopamine, a neurotransmitter associated with pleasure and reward in the brain. A dependency results as the brain begins to associate smoking or vaping with feeling good or finding relief from stress. The behavioral habits formed around smoking can add to the level of difficulty. Breaking this cycle requires not just physical withdrawal from nicotine but also a psychological battle to overcome these deeply ingrained associations.

The Challenge of Quitting

Due to the addictive properties of nicotine and the behavioral habits formed around smoking, the challenge is challenge, but people are able to stop smoking and vaping. The withdrawal symptoms they contend with can include irritability, nicotine cravings, difficulty concentrating, and an increased appetite. These physical symptoms peak within the first few days of quitting and gradually diminish over time, but the psychological urge to smoke can persist much longer. That's where finding some support can make a huge difference.

Numerous resources are available to help you manage withdrawal symptoms and reduce the urge to smoke. Here are some effective methods and tools that can support the process:

1. **Nicotine Replacement Therapies (NRTs)**
   - *Nicotine patches* deliver a steady dose of nicotine through the skin, helping to reduce withdrawal symptoms and nicotine cravings. By providing a consistent level of nicotine, patches also help break the habitual hand-to-mouth motion associated with smoking.
   - *Nicotine gum and lozenges* release nicotine into the bloodstream through the lining of the mouth, offering quick relief from nicotine cravings. These options appeal to the oral fixation of smoking, making it easier to manage the urge.
   - *Nicotine nasal sprays and inhalers* deliver nicotine through the nasal lining or lungs, providing rapid relief from intense nicotine cravings.

2. **Behavioral Therapy**
   - *Cognitive Behavioral Therapy* (CBT) helps individuals recognize and then change the thought patterns and behaviors that have supported their smoking. Whether conducted individually or in group settings, CBT provides people with tools to help better manage triggers and cravings.
   - *Motivational Interviewing* (MI) is designed to strengthen motivation and to resolve addictive behaviors by helping individuals explore their feelings about quitting. This technique is particularly effective in overcoming any ambivalence a person has about giving up smoking.
3. **Support Groups and Quitlines**
   - *Support groups* offer a sense of community and a shared understanding. Talking with others who are on their journey to be free of nicotine addiction can provide encouragement and valuable strategies.
   - *Quitlines* are telephone-based counseling services. Trained counselors offer personalized advice, resources, and emotional support. The National Quitline in the US (1-800-QUIT-NOW) offers a variety of free services.
4. **Healthy Lifestyle Changes**
   - *Exercise*: Regular physical activity can reduce both nicotine cravings and withdrawal symptoms. Exercise also improves mood, releases endorphins, and promotes overall health, making it easier to remain smoke-free.
   - *Healthy Diet*: A balanced diet rich in fruits, vegetables, and whole grains can help manage weight and stabilize mood during the quitting process. Drinking water and choosing healthy snacks can also reduce cravings.
5. **Stress Management Techniques**
   - *Mindfulness and meditation* promote relaxation, reduce stress, and help regulate emotions, all of which can reduce the urge to smoke.
   - *Deep breathing exercises* can calm the mind and body, providing a quick and effective way to manage cravings during stressful moments.

By combining these resources and strategies, individuals looking to quit smoking or vaping can increase their chances of success. It's important to remember that breaking away from the addiction is a process, and seeking help from healthcare professionals and support networks can make a significant difference. There is no safe level of smoking. Every cigarette avoided is a victory for your health and your future self will thank you.

EXCESSIVE SCREEN TIME

In today's digital age, screens have become an integral part of our lives. Smartphones and computers are constantly available and beckoning us to engage in a virtual world. This 24/7 connectivity comes with its share of drawbacks that affect both our physical and mental health in ways we're only beginning to understand.

Excessive screen time can take a toll on our eyes, leading to a condition known as digital eye strain. Symptoms include dryness, itchiness, and blurred vision, all resulting from staring at a screen for too long without giving our eyes a break. Furthermore, exposure to the blue light emitted by these devices, especially before bedtime, interferes with our natural sleep cycles. The blue light can suppress the production of melatonin, the hormone responsible for regulating sleep, making it harder for us to fall asleep and affecting the quality of our rest.

But the impact of screen time extends beyond our eyesight. Our physical health is also at risk due to the sedentary lifestyle that long hours of screen use often foster. Extended periods of sitting or lounging can lead to poor posture, causing neck and back pain, commonly referred to as "tech neck." This physical inactivity not only contributes to weight gain and obesity but also to an increased risk of developing related health issues such as diabetes and heart disease.

Excessive screen use also significantly affects mental health. Time spent on social media and other digital platforms can lead to feelings of loneliness, depression, and anxiety, particularly among teenagers. The constant exposure to the curated highlights of other people's lives can create unrealistic expectations and diminish self-esteem. For adolescents, whose brains are still developing, the allure of screens can be particularly addictive, making it difficult to disconnect and engage in real-life activities.

A few statistics highlight the urgency of addressing excessive screen time. Teens who spend more than five hours a day on electronic devices are significantly more likely to exhibit risk factors for depression and suicide compared to those who use screens for less than an hour. Children who exceed two hours of screen time daily are at a higher risk of being overweight or obese. And when it comes to sleep, those who engage with screens before bed are likely to experience longer sleep onset and disrupted sleep patterns.

Reducing screen time, therefore, becomes imperative to our health and well-being. Setting daily screen time limits and sticking to them can help us manage our digital consumption. Creating screen-free zones, particularly in bedrooms and dining areas, can encourage better sleep hygiene and foster richer family interactions. Offline activities that promote physical activity and creativity like sports, reading, or arts and crafts are fulfilling alternatives to screen time.

Parents and adults can lead by example. Our balanced screen habits and active participation in nondigital activities can encourage younger family members to do the same. That said, we adults are not immune to screen addiction. We can easily spend excessive time scrolling on smartphones, gaming, or spending time on any other digital platforms and as a result experience sleep issues, eye strain, and even mental health struggles like anxiety or depression. For our own well-being, we adults need to monitor our screen habits and take steps to limit our screen time. If you find yourself constantly drawn to your phone or gaming console, try taking regular breaks to engage in nondigital hobbies, like reading, exercising, or spending time outdoors.

Why not challenge yourself this weekend? Track your phone use and see if you can manage an afternoon or even a full day without it. Try replacing your screen time with a relaxing activity. Take a walk or catch up with a friend. If...*when*...you accept this challenge, note how you felt afterward. May this exercise help you realize that small changes can help reset your dependency on screens and significantly improve your overall well-being.

Of course screens aren't all bad. They undeniably serve as valuable resources for communication, learning, and entertainment, yet we must recognize and mitigate their potential negative impact. By being mindful of your screen time and implementing practical strategies like regular breaks or digital detoxes, you can improve both your physical and mental health, leading to a more balanced and fulfilling life.

Screen Time and Your Children

Too much screen time is becoming a significant concern for children's development, impacting mental, emotional, and physical well-being. A key worry is how screen time affects a child's capacity to stay focused and learn. In their world, the norm is flipping between apps and watching videos that move at lightning speed. Being accustomed to this level of constant stimulation, children find it challenging to concentrate on slower-paced activities that require more patience, such as reading a book or paying attention during lessons.

Moreover, the influence of screens on children's sleep patterns cannot be overstated. The blue light emitted by screens interferes with children's natural sleep cycles just as it does with adults. Children and adults alike can struggle to fall asleep and enjoy uninterrupted rest. Yet sleep is crucial for children: it supports both physical and brain development, ensuring they grow up healthy and strong.

Physically, an abundance of screen time promotes a sedentary lifestyle. With children spending hours in front of screens, they have less time for exercise and outdoor fun. The risk of obesity and associated health problems like heart disease increases. This shift away from active play to screen time is changing the very nature of childhood, impacting not only the children's physical health but also their social skills. We need to give our children opportunities to interact with their peers in a screen-free environment. There they will learn valuable lessons in cooperation, empathy, and conflict resolution, skills that are foundational for building relationships throughout life.

Emotionally, the effects of screen time are profound. Excessive use can cultivate feelings of isolation and sadness in children, particularly as they view the seemingly perfect lives of others on social media platforms. This comparison and the sense of missing out can have a significant impact on a child's self-esteem and overall happiness. In younger children, being habitually entertained by screens can lead to behavioral issues, such as tantrums and mood swings, when they're not engaged by digital content.

In essence, while screens have become an inescapable part of modern life, their impact on children's learning, health, social skills, and emotional well-being underscores the need for moderation. Finding a balance between screen time and other activities is crucial to ensuring that children develop into well-rounded, healthy individuals. These remarkable statistics illustrate the issues:

- **Teen Screen Time:** On average, teens spend more than 7 hours per day on screens for entertainment, and those 7 hours do not include screen time spent on schoolwork
- **Obesity:** Children who spend more than 2 hours a day on screens have a 30% higher risk of being overweight or obese compared to those who spend less time on screens.
- **Sleep Disruption:** 60% of adolescents who use screens right before bed report poor sleep quality when compared to 45% of those with minimal pre-sleep screen use.
- **Mental Health:** Compared to those who spend 1 hour a day, teens who spend 5 or more hours a day on electronic devices are 71% more likely to have one risk factor for suicide.
- **Physical Activity:** Only 1 in 3 children are physically active every day, and this decline is due in part to an increase in screen time.
- **Eye Strain:** More than 65% of Americans report symptoms of digital eye strain, such as dryness, irritation, and blurred vision, due to prolonged screen use.
- **Social Skills** At age 4, children who spend more time on screens at age 2 are more likely to have lower social and emotional development scores than their less-plugged-in peers.

Finding a Balance

Screens are here to stay, so finding a healthy balance between screen time and non-screen time is essential for our overall well-being. Encouraging kids to have a mix of screen-free playtime, physical activities, and opportunities to socialize with others in person can help mitigate the negative effects of too much screen time. Here are some strategies to help you find that balance:

1. **Set Clear Guidelines and Limits**
    - Establishing clear rules about screen time usage is crucial. Consider setting daily or weekly limits on the amount of time spent on screens; designating certain times of the day (during meals or an hour before bedtime) as screen-free; and ensuring that screen use doesn't interfere with important activities like homework, chores, and family time.

- Creating a family media plan can help set these boundaries and expectations. (Engaging the children in the conversation may facilitate their buy-in.) This plan should be flexible enough to accommodate the unexpected but strict enough to maintain a healthy routine.

2. **Encourage Physical Activity**
   - Physical activity is vital to children's health and development. Encourage kids to engage in regular physical activities such as participating in sports, going for walks or bike rides, taking dance classes, or simply playing outside. Physical activity not only promotes physical health but also helps reduce stress and improve mood.
   - Incorporate family activities that involve movement. Hike, play catch, or have dance-offs in the living room. Making exercise a fun and integral part of daily life can reduce the allure of screens.

3. **Promote Screen-Free Playtime**
   - Encourage creative and imaginative play that doesn't involve screens. Play with toys, draw, read books, or do some crafts. Screen-free playtime helps develop cognitive, social, and emotional skills.
   - Provide a variety of nondigital toys and materials that stimulate creativity and problem-solving. Board games, jigsaw puzzles, and outdoor games can be great alternatives to screen time.
   - Foster Social Interaction
   - Encourage children and teenagers to spend time with friends and family members in person. Social interaction like playdates, family gatherings, and community events is essential for developing communication and interpersonal skills.
   - Organize activities that promote teamwork and cooperation. The interactions that come with group sports, theatre productions, and collaborative projects help build strong social networks and may even reduce reliance on digital communication.

4. **Model Healthy Screen Use**
   - Children often emulate the behavior of the adults in their world. Parents and caregivers can set a positive example of healthy screen use by avoiding excessive screen time, prioritizing face-to-face interactions, and demonstrating a limited use of digital devices.

- Show children how to use screens for educational activities, research, and creative projects. Highlighting the constructive aspects of screen use can help children develop a more balanced relationship with technology.

5. **Designate Tech-Free Zones and Times**
    - Designate as tech-free zones specific areas in the home, such as bedrooms, dining areas, and outdoor spaces. This physical boundary between digital devices and personal or family time can foster a limited and healthier amount of screen time.
    - As mentioned above, establish tech-free times during the day. Mealtimes and the half-hour before bedtime can instead be used for relaxation, conversation, and unwinding without the distraction of screens.

6. **Encourage Responsible Digital Behavior**
    - Teach children responsible digital behavior. Help them understand the risks of excessive screen time, recognize the value of privacy, and be mindful of their digital footprint. Simply ask them, for example, to consider whether they are comfortable with what they share online being accessible for years to come.
    - Encourage open discussions about both the content they encounter online and how their digital interactions make them and others feel. Are they feeling connected or isolated? Empowered or anxious? Are their online words building others up or tearing them down? These conversations will help children develop critical thinking skills, make informed choices, and create a healthy, respectful online presence.

7. **Involve Kids in Decision-Making**
    - Involving kids in decisions about screen time can teach them how to manage their own screen use in a healthy way. Allowing children to have a say in setting screen time limits can increase their sense of responsibility and encourage ownership of their digital habits.
    - Encourage kids to reflect on their screen time usage and its impact on their daily life. This self-awareness can help them be more intentional about when and how to use screens.
    - Ensure Quality Sleep

- Limiting screen use, especially before bedtime, can help ensure that children get the sleep they need. Blue light from screens can interfere with the production of melatonin, the hormone responsible for regulating sleep.
- Create a bedtime routine that includes winding down without screens. Read a book, listen to calming music, or engage in quiet conversation to help signal to the body that it's time to sleep.

8. **Educational Screen Time**
    - Integrate educational and productive screen use even as you wisely seek to limit it. Encourage educational apps, documentaries, and interactive learning tools that can enhance knowledge and skills.
    - Balance entertainment and educational content to make screen time more enriching and purposeful.

CAFFEINE

Many of us love our morning coffee or tea. It's often the first thing we reach for to kick-start our day. Whether in an espresso, a latte, or, in the afternoon, a can of cola, caffeine plays a huge role in modern life, helping to boost our alertness and get or keep us going. In fact, over 80% of the world's population consumes a caffeinated product every day. It's no surprise, then, that caffeine has become deeply ingrained in our daily routines and culture. From catching up with friends at a coffee shop to sipping tea while we're at our desk, it's part of both our social and our work life.

As a doctor, though, I occasionally have patients ask if their caffeine intake might be causing health issues and it might. Caffeine can help us stay focused and alert, but it may also lead to problems if we consume it in excess or at the wrong time of day.

Coffee is the most popular source of caffeine for adults, with an estimated 2.25 billion cups consumed globally every day. The average intake among US adults is about 135 mg of caffeine per day, which is roughly equivalent to 1.5 cups of coffee. That morning cup might be what powers you through the start of your day, but overloading on caffeine throughout the day or reaching for a coffee late in the afternoon can come with some complications.

Caffeine can create a sense of fake alertness, making you feel more energized than you really are. While that might seem helpful in the moment, it can backfire at bedtime. You may find yourself wired, your heart racing, and your mind buzzing with anxiety or stress. For some people, caffeine can mean restless nights, interrupted sleep, and even feelings of burnout.

Energy Drinks and Caffeinated Beverages

Recent years have seen an increase in the consumption of energy drinks, particularly among young adults and teens. These beverages often contain high levels of caffeine, sometimes two to three times the amount found in a regular cup of coffee. A typical energy drink can contain between 80 mg and 300 mg of caffeine, with brands like Monster, Red Bull, and Rockstar leading the market.

The increasing popularity of these drinks has led to concerns about their impact on health, especially when consumed in large quantities or combined with other stimulants. Emergency room visits related to energy drink consumption have risen considerably, prompted by side effects ranging from jitteriness and rapid heart rate to more severe outcomes like heart palpitations or high blood pressure. Also popular among younger people, cola drinks can sneak up to 40 mg of caffeine per can into your diet. That amount may not seem like much, but multiple cans in a day add up, potentially leading to the same side effects of excessive caffeine consumption caused by coffee.

How Caffeine Can Mess with Sleep

Caffeine puts the brakes on a sleep chemical called adenosine that naturally occurs in your body and tells your brain it's time to wind down. When caffeine shows up, it blocks that signal, keeping you in a state of alertness. This trick can be super-helpful for shaking off sleepiness in the morning or giving you a boost when you're dragging in the middle of the day.

But drinking caffeine later in the day is particularly dicey because it messes with your sleep in a couple of big ways. First, caffeine can make it tough to fall asleep. Then, if you do manage to doze off, the quality of your sleep might take a hit because caffeine reduces the amount of deep, restorative sleep you get. You might wake up feeling like you didn't rest at all. Consuming caffeine too close to bedtime can lead to difficulties in falling asleep, to lighter sleep, and to lower quality sleep. Over time, not getting enough good sleep can make it hard to concentrate, affect your mood, and even weaken your immune system.

Jenna Cuts the Cord

> Jenna, a 36-year-old marketing executive, joked that coffee ran through her veins. But behind the humor was habit: five cups a day, plus an energy drink before afternoon meetings. Her sleep was erratic, her anxiety spiked, and her stomach felt like it was always churning.
>
> When she started waking up feeling exhausted despite eight hours in bed, she knew something had to give. Her doctor suggested tracking her intake and tapering gradually. Jenna replaced her second coffee with green tea, then swapped her afternoon energy drink for sparkling water with lemon.
>
> She also started stretching at 2 p.m. instead of refilling her mug, and focused on eating more whole foods to steady her energy. Within three weeks, she was down to one small cup in the morning and for the first time in years, she wasn't wired or tired.
>
> Kicking caffeine didn't mean giving up productivity. For Jenna, it meant finally feeling in control.

The Best Time for Caffeine

The best time of day to stop drinking caffeine depends on several factors, including your sensitivity to caffeine, your typical caffeine consumption, and your sleep schedule. Generally, the recommendation is to stop drinking caffeine at least 6 to 8 hours before bedtime to ensure it doesn't interfere with your sleep. For the average adult, caffeine has a half-life of about 3 to 5 hours, which means that half of the caffeine you consume is still in your system after 3 to 5 hours. Some people take longer to metabolize caffeine, up to 8 hours or more.

Clearly, people have different levels of sensitivity to caffeine. Some individuals may metabolize caffeine quickly and can tolerate consuming it closer to bedtime; other people are more sensitive and need a longer window to avoid sleep disturbances. In general, try to stop consuming caffeine at least 6 to 8 hours before you plan to go to bed. For example, if you aim to go to bed at 10 p.m., it would be best to avoid caffeine after 2 p.m. Pay attention to how caffeine affects your sleep. If you notice that you have trouble falling asleep or you experience restless sleep, consider moving your caffeine cutoff time to earlier in the day. If you consume a lot of caffeine, try gradually reducing your intake rather than stopping abruptly. Then you'll avoid withdrawal symptoms such as headaches or irritability.

Switching to decaffeinated versions of coffee or herbal tea in the afternoon and evening can help you enjoy the taste without the potential sleep disruption. Herbal teas are generally caffeine-free and can be a good alternative for an evening beverage. Additionally, drinking water can help you stay hydrated and avoid the potential sleep disruption that caffeine can cause. By finding the right balance and timing for your caffeine consumption, you can enjoy the benefits of caffeine and minimize its impact on your sleep and overall well-being.

The Impact of Caffeine on Your Neurotransmitters

In addition to affecting adenosine, caffeine also impacts how other neurotransmitters work in your brain. Caffeine, for instance, gives a nudge to dopamine, the feel-good chemical, which is why that first sip of coffee can be so satisfying. Caffeine also amps up norepinephrine, which can make you feel more awake and alert. Then acetylcholine, involved in focus and learning, gets a boost from caffeine's stimulating effects. Caffeine can even influence the mood-regulator serotonin, although this connection is a bit more indirect.

Understanding this intricate dance of neurotransmitters helps explain why caffeine can so profoundly affect our mood, energy, and alertness and why too much caffeine can lead to feeling jittery or anxious. When we find the right amount of caffeine, we can keep our mind and body in harmony.

EATING MORE THAN WE NEED

Consistent overeating can result in serious health issues, as is very evident in the Western world. According to data from the CDC, around 42.4% of adults in the United States are considered obese. Even more concerning, 19.3% of US children and adolescents are obese, and that percentage translates to about 14.4 million young people. The World Health Organization reports that obesity worldwide has nearly tripled since 1975.

Poor eating habits among them, overeating are a major factor in the development of chronic diseases such as heart disease, type 2 diabetes, and some cancers. Roughly 34.2 million Americans just over 1 in 10 have diabetes, and the majority of adult cases are type 2, largely influenced by diet and obesity. People who are obese have an increased risk for heart disease, and obesity is linked to about one in every four deaths from heart disease.

Let's look in detail at the impact of eating more than we need.

When we consume more food than our body needs, our digestive system has to work overtime, leading to such discomfort as bloating and indigestion. The pancreas and liver also bear a heavy load: they need to produce enough enzymes and bile to break down the excess food. Acid reflux, where stomach acid irritates the esophagus, can result, meaning more discomfort and potential long-term damage. This continuous strain can lead to chronic conditions that affect the organs of the digestive system. Also, when we consume more food than our body needs, the excess calories are stored as fat. The body converts surplus nutrients whether fats, carbohydrates, or proteins into triglycerides that are stored in fat cells. This increased body fat affects heart health by elevating blood cholesterol and boosting triglyceride levels. These changes can lead to arteries to narrow and harden (atherosclerosis), significantly increasing the risk of heart disease. High blood pressure, a common consequence of obesity, further exacerbates the risk of cardiovascular issues.

Furthermore, regular overeating can disrupt metabolic processes and lead to insulin resistance: cells in muscles, fat, and the liver stop responding well to insulin. Their hindered ability to take up glucose from the blood can elevate blood glucose levels and eventually lead to type 2 diabetes.

The liver is particularly affected by excessive eating, especially the ingestion of too much high-fat and high-sugar food. Nonalcoholic fatty liver disease (NAFLD) can occur as fat accumulates in liver cells. Affecting about 25% of the global population, NAFLD can progress to more severe liver damage such as nonalcoholic steatohepatitis (NASH), fibrosis, and cirrhosis.

Overeating can also impact brain function by altering levels of dopamine, the neurotransmitter responsible for reward and pleasure. This alteration can create a cycle of cravings and dependency similar to what is found with addictive behaviors. Moreover, poor dietary habits can lead to inflammation that may negatively impact cognitive function over time.

Consuming large amounts of food, particularly in the evening, can disrupt sleep quality by causing physical discomfort and indigestion. Research shows that high-fat diets are particularly detrimental, reducing both sleep duration and quality as well as exacerbating sleep apnea. (Over 50% of obese individuals suffer from sleep apnea.) Poor sleep can affect overall health and impair immune function, cognitive performance, and mood.

Recognizing if you are overeating isn't always hard: you probably already have a sense if your clothes are fitting tighter, if you feel sluggish, or if you feel more out of shape than before. Or maybe you're experiencing regular discomfort after meals, or you find yourself reaching for snacks out of habit rather than hunger. If any of this sounds familiar, know that there's plenty you can do to support your health and make positive changes. By being mindful of your portions, choosing nutrient-rich foods, and paying attention to hunger cues, you can adopt sustainable habits that will improve your well-being and enhance your quality of life.

Metabolic Syndrome

Unhealthy eating habits can lead to a range of health issues, one of the most significant being metabolic syndrome. Not a disease itself, metabolic syndrome is a group of risk factors high blood pressure, high blood sugar, unhealthy cholesterol levels, and abdominal fat that increase the risk of heart disease, stroke, and diabetes.

When we consume foods high in fats, sugars, and calories, our body must work hard to process it all. Foods high in simple carbohydrates, such as white bread, sugary drinks, and snacks, can cause blood sugar levels to spike rapidly. In response, the pancreas releases insulin, a hormone that helps cells absorb glucose (sugar) from the bloodstream and use it for energy. Over time, if the body is consistently flooded with large amounts of sugar, the cells can become less sensitive to insulin. This condition, known as insulin resistance, is a key component of metabolic syndrome. According to the American Heart Association, about 1 in 3 adults in the United States have metabolic syndrome, making it a widespread health concern with long-term consequences if it isn't addressed.

As insulin resistance develops, the body's ability to regulate blood sugar levels diminishes, leading to higher blood sugar levels and, if the pattern continues, eventually type 2 diabetes. Additionally, diets high in saturated and trans fats can lead to increases in harmful LDL cholesterol, which accumulates in the arteries and increases the risk of heart attacks and strokes. Saturated and trans fats can also contribute to the development of abdominal fat, another risk factor for metabolic syndrome.

The excessive intake of salty and high-fat foods can raise blood pressure, putting additional strain on the heart and vascular system. High blood pressure (hypertension) is another risk factor associated with metabolic syndrome. To summarize, the following conditions put a person at significant risk for serious health issues:

1. **High Blood Sugar:** Diets rich in simple sugars and refined carbs lead to frequent spikes in blood sugar and insulin levels. Over time, this pattern can lead to insulin resistance.
2. **Abdominal Obesity:** Consuming more calories than the body can use means fat accumulation. Fat stored around the abdomen is particularly dangerous because it secretes hormones and substances that can trigger whole-body inflammation.
3. **Unhealthy Cholesterol Levels:** Eating foods high in saturated and trans fats can increase bad cholesterol (LDL) and decrease good cholesterol (HDL), contributing to the buildup of fatty deposits in arteries.
4. **High Blood Pressure:** Excessive salt intake can cause the body to retain water, and that raises blood pressure. High-fat diets can also contribute to hardened arteries, making it harder for the heart to pump blood effectively.

Taking Steps Toward Healthy Eating

You have the power to take control of your eating habits, and you can start that transformation today. Every small step can make a difference by helping to reverse conditions like insulin resistance and by reducing the risk of other health issues. Being mindful and deliberate with your food choices, you'll be improving your overall well-being and prescribing for yourself a healthier future.

Mindful Eating

When you eat, whether a meal or a snack, focus on the flavor, texture, and aroma of your food. By paying close attention to the experience of eating, you become more attuned to your body's hunger and fullness signals, and you may find yourself feeling satisfied with smaller portions. Avoid distractions during meals. Watching TV or using your phone while you have dinner can lead to mindless overeating. You can reset your relationship with food simply by paying attention to the eating experience.

Choose a Balanced Diet

A balanced diet ensures that you are consuming the variety of nutrients necessary for maintaining health. Structuring your meals to include a diverse range of foods helps cover the spectrum of your body's needs. Aim to fill half your plate with vegetables and fruits that are rich in essential vitamins, minerals, and fiber. Place in a quarter of the plate lean proteins such as eggs, chicken, fish, legumes, or tofu to support muscle repair and growth. The remaining quarter of the plate is for whole grains like brown rice, whole wheat pasta, or potatoes that provide fiber and sustained energy.

Foods high in added sugar and unhealthy fat often found in processed snacks, baked goods, and fast food can contribute to weight gain and reduce the quality of your diet. Try to minimize consumption of such foods. Instead, choose whole foods with natural ingredients and minimal additives.

Establishing a routine of regular, spaced-out meals can help stabilize blood sugar levels and make managing hunger easier. Skipping meals often leads to excessive hunger that increases the likelihood of overeating later in the day. Instead, aim to eat at consistent times throughout the day. If you can't avoid long gaps between meals, find healthy snacks that contain protein or vegetables, such as a handful of nuts, hummus with carrot sticks, or a boiled egg. These options will help keep you satisfied without spiking your blood sugar.

Drink Plenty of Water

In addition to being vital for overall health, proper hydration can aid in appetite control because feeling hungry is often a sign of dehydration. Before reaching for a snack, drink a glass of water and wait a few minutes. You may find that hydration was all you needed. Aim to drink at least eight glasses of water a day and more if you're active or if the weather is hot.

Cook at Home

Cooking at home puts you in control of your diet. Homemade meals tend to be healthier than take-out and restaurant meals because you can choose whole ingredients and cook in ways that preserve nutrients but limit fat and salt. Experiment with herbs and spices to flavor your dishes instead of relying on heavy sauces or seasonings.

Read Labels

Becoming familiar with nutritional labels is an essential skill for making informed food choices. Look for products that are low in sugar, sodium, and saturated fats but high in fiber and nutrients. Be mindful of the serving sizes (indicated on the packaging) to avoid consuming more than you intend or need.

Pay Attention to Portion Control

Managing portion sizes can significantly affect your calorie intake. Using smaller plates, bowls, and utensils can help you take smaller portions. When eating out, consider sharing a meal or taking half to go. You'll also be preventing overeating when you listen to your body and stop eating when you're comfortably full.

Calorie Intake vs Expenditure

Understanding the balance between calorie intake and calorie expenditure is essential to maintaining a healthy weight and preventing obesity-related health issues. *Calorie intake* refers to the energy consumed through food and drink. An individual's caloric needs vary based on factors like age, gender, size, and level of physical activity. High-calorie foods, especially those rich in fats and sugars, can lead to excess calorie intake.

Calorie expenditure refers to the energy the body uses to maintain basic bodily functions at rest (known as *basal metabolic rate*) plus the energy used during physical activity. For most adults, the basal metabolic rate is around 1,000 to 1,300 calories per day. When factoring in routine activities such as standing, walking, and exercise, the total daily energy expenditure can range from 1,800 to 2,500 calories, depending on activity level.

According to the American Heart Association, an average adult woman should consume 1,800 to 2,200 calories per day, and an average adult man should consume 2,400 to 3,000 calories per day, depending on activity level. Consuming more calories than the body expends leads to weight gain. Over time, this consistent excess can cause obesity. Conversely, ensuring that calorie intake matches or is less than expenditure can prevent weight gain or support weight loss, respectively. Strategies for achieving this balance include adopting a diet rich in vegetables, fruits, lean proteins, and whole grains and at the same time avoiding calorie-dense, nutrition-poor foods. Regular physical activity is also crucial. In addition to increasing the number of calories burned, being active boosts metabolism and muscle mass, further enhancing caloric burn even when we're at rest. Finally, be more mindful of food intake: reading nutritional labels, controlling portion sizes, and avoiding mindless eating can significantly help you manage calorie intake.

Balancing calorie intake and expenditure is more than avoiding weight gain or losing weight; it's about enhancing overall health and longevity. A consistently healthy diet reduces the risk of metabolic disorders, improves cardiac health, and sustains higher energy levels. Becoming educated about the caloric content of foods and the energy expenditure of different activities can empower individuals to make informed choices about their diet and activity levels, thus promoting a healthier lifestyle.

Avoid Crash Diets; Aim for Consistency

Fad or crash diets like extremely low-carbohydrate diets, juice cleanses, or diets that involve eating only one specific type of food, such as grapefruit or cabbage soup often promise quick weight loss and even other health benefits. The initial rapid weight loss, usually achieved by restricting certain types of foods or drastically cutting calories, may be appealing, but these diets are typically unsustainable, and some can be harmful in the long run.

The primary downside of fad diets is that they often lack nutritional balance. With the exclusion of key food groups, we risk deficiencies in essential nutrients, which can lead to health problems over time. Extremely low-carb or high-protein diets, for instance, can strain the kidneys and liver and may cause a significant loss of minerals, leading to bone density issues and other metabolic changes. Moreover, a high proportion of the weight lost by someone trying a fad diet is often due to the loss of water and muscle mass, not much fat.

Consistent eating habits and mindful eating, on the other hand, offer a more sustainable and healthier approach to achieving and maintaining a healthy weight. Mindful eating involves paying attention to the body's hunger and fullness cues, a focus that can help prevent overeating. It also encourages awareness of the sensory experience of eating and fosters a deeper connection with food choices, promoting satisfaction and enjoyment in meals.

Maintaining a balanced diet that includes a variety of nutrients from all food groups is an important aspect of consistent and healthy eating. Nutrition experts agree that incorporating a wide range of food including vegetables, fruits, whole grains, lean proteins, and healthy fats provides the body with a comprehensive array of nutrients essential for optimal functioning. This approach supports long-term health benefits, including maintained weight loss, a stable weight, improved metabolic fitness, and reduced risk of chronic diseases such as diabetes, heart disease, and certain cancers. Studies show that people who eat a balanced diet with a consistent approach are more likely to maintain their weight loss and enjoy improved health markers.

Overall, while fad diets may offer quick results, they are often associated with health risks and high amounts of regained weight. Adopting consistent eating habits and practicing mindful eating are much more effective for maintaining a healthy weight and promoting overall well-being. This approach ensures that the body gets what it needs to function properly and sustainably over the long term, making it a far better choice than the latest diet trend.

Don't Just Sit There (Or Why Inactivity Is Bad for You)

Inactivity, particularly prolonged sitting, poses significant health risks and is increasingly recognized as a serious public health concern. Often referred to as "the new smoking," sedentary behavior is linked to a myriad of health problems that can have profound implications on long-term wellness.

To be specific, a sedentary lifestyle increases the risk of obesity, type 2 diabetes, cardiovascular disease, cancer, and other chronic diseases. When we sit for extended periods, our metabolism slows down, reducing the rate at which the body burns calories and processes sugar. Depending on our calorie intake, this reduced metabolic rate can lead to weight gain and associated health issues like high blood pressure, high cholesterol, and insulin resistance, which is a precursor to diabetes.

Prolonged sitting also has detrimental effects on the musculoskeletal system. Muscles and bones can weaken, and the lack of movement reduces blood flow, which can cause issues like deep vein thrombosis in the legs. Extended periods of inactivity can also contribute to poor posture and back pain due to the strain placed on the spine and neck from sitting in one position.

Excessive sedentary behavior can also impact mental health. Inactivity is associated with an increased risk of experiencing anxiety and depression. In contrast, physical activity has been shown to improve mood and energy levels by releasing endorphins, the body's natural stress-fighters.

Combating the negative effects of inactivity doesn't necessarily require intense exercise, though. Integrating simple forms of movement throughout the day can significantly reduce health risks. Here are some effective strategies:

1. **Take Short, Frequent Breaks:** Break up any long periods of sitting by standing or walking around for a few minutes every hour. Even short bursts of activity like stretching or walking to get some water can improve circulation and muscle activity.
2. **Work from a Standing Desk:** Alternating between sitting and standing throughout the day can help reduce the risks associated with prolonged sedentary behavior. If a standing desk isn't available, find a high counter or use a stack of books to elevate a laptop.
3. **Schedule Active Meetings:** Whenever possible, conduct meetings on the go. Walking meetings not only break the sedentary cycle but can also boost creativity and engagement.
4. **Set Reminders to Move:** Use a smartphone app or alarm to set reminders to stand up and move. Regular reminders can help incorporate into a sedentary routine the healthy habit of moving.
5. **Integrate Exercise into Everyday Activities:** Simple changes like taking the stairs instead of the elevator, parking farther away from the store entrance, stretching during work breaks, or doing light exercises while watching TV can increase the level of daily physical activity.

Be Aware: Sitting Is the New Smoking

Smoking was once widely accepted as harmless, and it became a societal norm.

Likewise, prolonged sitting has quietly become the norm in our modern, screen-dominated world. But like cigarettes, a sedentary lifestyle hides serious health risks. The dangers of staying sedentary, ranging from heart disease to obesity, are not unlike the risks once associated with smoking.

Here's where you hold the power to change. You don't need a prescription or a medical intervention to break free from the habits that keep you sedentary. Just as a reduced rate of smoking has brought a remarkable public health turnaround, we can transform our health by recognizing the risks of prolonged sitting and embracing more movement in our daily life.

The truth is, the steps to change are simple, and you are totally in control. Whether you choose to stand up during phone calls, walk during breaks, or set daily movement goals, these small but intentional efforts can lead to a significant improvement in your health. By incorporating more activity into your routine, you're not only reducing health risks but also reclaiming your vitality, energy, and long-term well-being.

In an age where we often rely on medication to manage ailments, it's empowering to know that movement is one of the best prescriptions you can give yourself. The choice is yours, and every interruption of your sedentary routine counts as a step toward a healthier, more fulfilling life. Break the chains of inactivity and embrace the power you have to healthy changes for your body and mind.

Personal Empowerment

I hope this chapter has not only helped you recognize your ability to influence your health and life outcomes positively but also empowered you to act. I hope you are seeing yourself as the primary agent of change and finding that a powerful and liberating perspective. You have the capacity to make choices that significantly impact your well-being, and acknowledging this truth is the first step toward breaking unhealthy habits and making positive and lasting changes.

That said, another truth is, making lifestyle changes can be challenging. Habits, especially those related to addictive behaviors like smoking, alcohol consumption, and unhealthy eating, are often deeply ingrained. They may also have served as coping mechanisms or sources of comfort during stressful times, making the process of changing them more complex and daunting.

These unhealthy behaviors might also be tied to social routines and personal identities, which adds another layer of difficulty to altering them. But challenging and difficult doesn't mean impossible.

Also, keep in mind that the journey toward change is rarely linear. It often involves setbacks and challenges that test one's resolve. Acknowledging and preparing for these potential obstacles is crucial. So is understanding that any setbacks you might encounter aren't failures but part of the learning process that can provide valuable insight into your behaviors and their triggers.

Here are a few strategies for successfully navigating the difficulties of changing your behaviors:

1. **Set Clear, Achievable, and Measurable Goals**: Start small with manageable changes so you build confidence and momentum. Even tiny wins will motivate you to work toward greater progress.
2. **Seek Support**: Lean on friends, call on family, or find support groups who understand the challenges you face and can offer encouragement and accountability.
3. **Explore Healthy Alternatives**: Replace unhealthy habits with constructive activities. Swap a night at the bar for a walk in the park with friends or some other relaxing activity that you enjoy.
4. **Track and Celebrate Your Progress**: Keep a journal or log where you can note your improvements. Seeing how far you've come can boost morale and keep you motivated.
5. **Extend Compassion to Yourself**: Change takes time. Be patient and kind to yourself, especially during setbacks. Extending yourself compassion will help you stay on track rather than getting bogged down in discouragement.
6. **Establish a Routine**: Building a daily routine makes it easier to adopt healthier habits and maintain them over time. Consistency is key.
7. **Visualize Success**: Spend a few minutes each day picturing yourself achieving your goals. This mental image reinforces motivation and commitment.
8. **Reward Yourself**: Celebrate your successes no matter how small. Rewards can be simple and inexpensive, perhaps taking a leisurely bath or spending time on a hobby.
9. **Learn from Setbacks**: Setbacks are part of the process, so view them as valuable learning experiences instead of failures. Figure out what went wrong, adjust your strategy, and take the next step forward.

The challenges of changing your behaviors are real, but so is your personal power to act. You have the power and ability to make transformative choices. Being realistic and optimistic enhances the likelihood that you'll make lasting improvements in your health and experience a more fulfilling, self-directed life overall. By taking small steps, you can make sustainable changes that empower you to take charge of your well-being and thrive. You can be your own prescription for better health.

10 Ways to Break Free from Unhealthy Habits

1. Identify Your Triggers

Every habit has a trigger a set of circumstances, an emotion, a memory that activates it. Recognizing your triggers is the first step in taking control of unhealthy habits.

Ask yourself:

- Do I smoke after meals or when I'm stressed?
- Do I binge-eat when I'm alone or bored?
- Do I scroll endlessly on my phone when I'm anxious?

Once you identify your triggers, respond to them with a healthier response. If stress triggers smoking, take a five-minute walk instead. If boredom leads to snacking, pick up a book or call a friend.

2. Set Clear, Achievable Goals

Saying, "I want to quit smoking" is not enough. Instead, make your goal specific, measurable, and realistic.

- Instead of "I will stop drinking," try "I will only drink on weekends for the next 30 days."
- Instead of "I will stop snacking," try "Every afternoon I will replace an unhealthy snack with a healthy option."

The clearer your goal, the more likely you are to stay on track until you reach it.

3. Start Small, Win Big

Trying to break an unhealthy habit can feel overwhelming. Instead of going cold turkey, focus on small, manageable steps that will move you toward your goal.

- If you want to cut back on alcohol, start with alcohol-free weekdays.
- If you want to stop mindlessly scrolling on your phone, set a timer for 30 minutes max.
- If you want to quit smoking, first cut down your smoking by one cigarette per day.

Small wins build momentum and lead to lasting change.

4. Replace the Habit Instead of Just Stopping

Your brain hates giving things up. So instead of focusing on what you're removing, focus on what you're adding.

- Chew gum, sip water, or do some deep breathing instead of smoking.
- Swap junk food for high-protein snacks to help avoid overeating.
- To cut down on screen time, replace a TV episode with a walk or favorite creative activity.

When you give your brain something new and better, it will let go of the old unhealthy habit more easily.

5. Use Technology to Your Advantage

Your phone can be part of the problem—or part of the solution. Let habit-tracking apps hold you accountable to reaching your goals.

- Download a quit-smoking app to track your progress.
- Set screen-time limits to avoid social media addiction.
- Try using a food journal app to cut back on overeating.

Progress you can see is progress you will stick to.

6. Surround Yourself with Support, Not Temptation

The people you spend time with affect your habits. If your environment is filled with triggers, breaking free of bad behaviors will be harder.

- Let friends and family know about your goal.
- Join a support group or find a mentor who has already reached the goal you've set for yourself.
- Remove temptation: get junk food out of the house, turn off the Netflix autoplay, and put your e-cigarette in a hard-to-reach spot.

You don't have to break free from unhealthy habits alone. Find a support system.

7. Learn to De-Stress Without Turning to an Unhealthy Habit

Most unhealthy habits are a response to stress. If you don't find a new way to cope, the habit will creep back in.

Instead of reaching for an unhealthy habit:

- Take five deep breaths.
- Go for a 10-minute walk.
- Listen to music or a podcast.

When you teach your body to relax in new ways, your cravings lose their power.

8. Celebrate Small Wins (They Matter More Than You Think!)

Every step in the right direction counts. Acknowledge progress, no matter how small.

- You quit smoking for three days? That's a win.
- You didn't do any late-night snacking this evening? That's a win.
- You reduced your screen time by 30 minutes today? Another win.

Celebrating your progress will keep you motivated.

9. Prepare for Setbacks Because They Will Happen

Setbacks are part of the process, and everyone experiences them. Instead of giving up, figure out a few things:

- What triggered this setback?
- How can I adjust my strategy?
- What will I do differently next time?

Treat setbacks as learning experiences, not failures.

10. Track Progress and Stay Accountable

Tracking your progress leads to success. So keep a journal, use an app, or write on a calendar.

- Keep track of how many days you go without engaging in a favorite unhealthy habit.
- Write down how you feel when you aren't indulging in an unhealthy habit: Are you sleeping better? Do you have more energy? Are you feeling less stressed?
- Celebrate each milestone: one week, one month, 90 days.

Your Action Plan for Breaking Free from Unhealthy Habits

Transformation happens when you act. Use this section to identify patterns, track your progress, and build momentum as you break free from unhealthy habits.

1. Identify Your Habit Triggers

Before you can break a habit, you need to understand what triggers it. Take a moment to reflect on when, where, and why you engage in this habit.

Write down the habit you want to change:

_____

What triggers this habit? (Check all that apply.)

☐ Stress or anxiety

☐ Boredom

☐ Social pressure

☐ Certain people or environments

☐ Specific times of day

☐ Emotional eating or drinking

☐ Other: _____

Instead of falling back into your unhealthy habit, what can you do when you feel triggered?

Here's an example: Instead of stress-eating, I will drink a glass of water and go for a short walk.

2. Set a Clear, Achievable Goal

A vague goal like "I want to stop drinking" is hard to measure. Instead, make your goal specific, measurable, and realistic.

- **Rewrite your goal in a clear, measurable way:**

Example: "For the next 30 days I will only drink alcohol on weekends."

3. Replace an Unhealthy Habit with Something Better

Your brain needs an alternative reward to make quitting easier.

What can you replace your unhealthy habit with? (Check all that apply.)

☐ Swap smoking for deep breathing or chewing gum.

☐ Replace late-night snacking with a mug of herbal tea or a good book.

☐ Substitute mindless scrolling with a short walk or a book.

☐ Other: _____

Action Step: Write down one replacement habit you will start today:

4. Create a Support Plan

You don't have to break this unhealthy habit alone. Ask others to hold you accountable.

Who will be your accountability partner?

Name one person you can check in with about your progress.

Join a community for support (if applicable):

☐ A support group

☐ An online forum

☐ A coach or therapist

☐ A trusted friend or family member

5. Prepare for Setbacks

Setbacks don't mean failure; they're simply opportunities to learn. The key is having a plan for when they happen.

What might cause you to slip up? (Check all that apply)

- ☐ Social events with drinking or smoking
- ☐ Stressful situations
- ☐ Lack of motivation
- ☐ Peer pressure
- ☐ Boredom
- ☐ Other: _____

What will you do if you slip up?

Example: If I overeat at night, I won't beat myself up. Instead, I'll focus on making the next meal a healthy one.

6. Track Your Progress

Tracking your progress keeps you motivated.

For the next seven days, track your progress. At the end of each day, note whether you avoided the habit, you had a small slip but recovered, or you fully engaged in the habit and then how you felt afterward. What helped you avoid the habit? What pressure led to the small slip or full engagement?

Day 1:
_____

Day 2:
_____

Day 3:

Day 4:

Day 5:

Day 6:

Day 7:

7. Celebrate Small Wins

Recognizing your progress keeps you motivated.

What is one small victory you've had this week?

Example: I cut my screen time by 30 minutes per day.

How will you reward yourself for hitting a milestone?

Example: If I go seven days without late-night snacking, I will treat myself to a massage.

PART III
WHOLE HEALTH FOR EVERYONE

CHAPTER 7

THE POWER OF PREVENTION:

BUILDING A HEALTHIER TOMORROW

R onnie grew up in a small town, the youngest of five siblings in a close-knit family. Known for his vibrant personality and infectious laughter, he excelled in drama and thrived in various avenues of community service. After studying communications in college, he married a nursing student named Sarah. They built a loving home in the suburbs and raised three children. Ronnie owned a jewelry store, and his career flourished thanks to his natural charisma. Despite having been diagnosed with diabetes and high blood pressure when he was in his mid-forties, he often dismissed the severity of his conditions and continued to live life with unwavering optimism.

With his infectious laugh and legendary stories, Ronnie was once the life of every party. But as time passed, his uncontrolled diabetes and blood pressure caused his health to decline. Those conditions, which he initially dismissed, eventually took a toll on him, both physically and emotionally. The sparkle in his eyes dimmed when he lost sight in his right eye, and his heart, once so full of life, stopped beating on multiple occasions.

As Ronnie's health was crumbling, the COVID-19 pandemic, merciless and unyielding, swept through the world. Among its countless victims was Ronnie's wife. Sarah's passing meant the loss of her lifelong companionship and the cruel unveiling of his creeping dementia. Without her by his side to subtly cover for his forgetfulness or to gently steer conversations when he got lost in them, Ronnie's mental state became painfully apparent to everyone around him, especially to his children. His decline into dementia was heart-wrenching. He became a shell of the man he used to be, lost in the fog of his own mind.

Ronnie's story marked by laughter, love, loss, and dementia's relentless march reminds us of life's fragility and the cruel toll we may pay if we neglect our health. In the end, Ronnie's legacy was not just in the stories he had told but also in the lessons his life offered about the preciousness of health, the impact of its loss, and the enduring strength of family love through the darkest times. His memory calls us to cherish every moment, to hold our loved ones close, and to courageously confront the challenges of health and aging as they arise. Too many people lose the quality of their later years to preventable health issues. What can we do to protect our health and preserve our well-being for as long as possible? In this chapter, we'll explore steps you can take today to safeguard your future and to live your life to the fullest.

Your Quality of Life

Preventative health is not merely about avoiding illness; it's about optimizing your quality of life and empowering you to lead a fuller, more active life. Taking charge of your health is one of the most significant decisions you can make in your lifetime. The empowering act of self-care not only enhances your quality of life but can also extend it. The path of preventative health is paved with small, daily choices that together have a life-changing impact over time. This journey does not require drastic changes it requires committment. Taking charge of your health means making informed decisions that enhance your well-being now and into the future.

Your Health, Your Responsibility

Your health is arguably your most valuable asset, so be proactive in your taking care of it. Decide to integrate simple, preventative health measures into your lifestyle and then do it! Your journey will be unique to you, and it begins with your recognition that you have the ability and the power to protect and even improve your health. Remember that every step you take is a step toward a healthier you.

Protect Your Health

Preventative health is all about taking steps now to avoid getting sick later. You put up a strong, protective fence around your health to keep out potential illnesses and avoid health problems. This approach focuses you on doing things today that will help you stay healthy in the future. These actions can include the following:

- Get only the essential vaccines
- Eat healthy foods.
- Exercise regularly.
- Go in for regular checkups and screenings.

Chronic diseases like heart disease, diabetes, and mental health conditions manifest as more than just medical issues. Patients diagnosed with a chronic disease face relentless challenges that weigh them down, lower their quality of life, and often requiring lifelong management. Chronic diseases also impact financial well-being. In fact, most healthcare dollars in the US, 90% of our overwhelming $4.1 trillion annual total, are spent on chronic diseases.

But significant drivers of these chronic and debilitating health conditions are many of the lifestyle choices we make like smoking, poor nutrition, inactivity, and excessive alcohol use. With 42% of adults and 20% of children in the US affected by obesity, the risks for heart disease, diabetes, and other long-term health problems are incredibly high. Arthritis, Alzheimer's, and even dental issues like untreated cavities can erode the richness of life. But we aren't sentenced to sitting around waiting for poor health to strike. The good news is, it's never too late to start taking action.

No matter the current state of your health, simple lifestyle changes like staying active, eating nutritious foods, and cutting back on tobacco and alcohol can reduce your risk of chronic conditions and illnesses as well as improve your overall well-being. Your everyday choices are powerful. By making small, consistent changes, you can positively impact your future health and protect yourself from many of the chronic conditions that millions of people are dealing with today.

Consider these benefits of taking action today:

1. **You Stay Active:** When you keep diseases at bay, you can enjoy a more active, vibrant life.
2. **You Lower Your Health Costs:** Prevention will save you money in the long run by reducing the need for medical treatments, some of which can be very expensive.
3. **You Get Treated Earlier:** Regular screenings can catch health issues early when they're often easier to treat.
4. **You Have a Longer, Healthier Life:** Preventative care can help you live a longer, healthier life, giving you more time with friends and family.

Myth Buster

Being proactive about your health sounds simple, right? So why aren't more people pursuing preventative healthcare? Maybe too many have bought into some of the common myths debunked below. The corresponding facts will encourage you to make informed decisions that can lead to a healthier, happier life.

Preventative Care: Myths vs. Facts

Myth: "Preventative care is expensive."

Fact: Many preventative measures, like exercising and eating well, cost very little and will save you money on healthcare in the long run. Also, some insurance plans cover preventative services at no extra charge.

Myth: "I'm young and healthy, so I don't need preventative care."

Fact: Everyone, regardless of age, benefits from preventative health measures. Vaccinations and regular checkups are important at every age, and healthy habits formed early on and then maintained can ensure a longer, healthier life.

Myth: "If I feel fine, I don't need to see a doctor."

Fact: Some serious health conditions don't show symptoms in their early stages. Regular checkups catch these conditions early when treatment can be more effective.

Myth: "Preventative care doesn't really make a difference."

Fact: Research shows that preventative health measures, like screenings, vaccinations, and lifestyle changes, significantly reduce the risk of many common diseases, such as diabetes, heart disease, and even certain cancers.

Vaccinations: The First Line of Defense

Key to prevention, vaccinations stand as the frontline warriors in the battle against infectious diseases. They work by training your immune system to recognize and combat viruses and bacteria before they can cause illness. The global eradication of smallpox and the near elimination of polio highlight the unparalleled success of vaccines.

Staying up-to-date with vaccinations is just as essential for adults as it is for children. Annual flu shots, COVID boosters, tetanus updates, and vaccines for shingles and pneumococcal disease are crucial parts of preventative care for the average adult. By following recommended vaccination schedules, we do more than protect ourselves; we also contribute to community-wide herd immunity, helping to reduce the spread of infectious diseases and protecting the most vulnerable among us.

Go for Regular Screening

With vaccines serving as the frontline soldiers, screenings act as vigilant sentinels, quietly detecting signs of disease even before symptoms appear. These preventative measures are crucial for early diagnosis, and catching certain cancers early can significantly improve the outcome.

- **Breast Cancer**: Regular mammograms are essential to detecting breast cancer in its early and most treatable stages. The life-saving potential of a mammogram is worth the brief discomfort of the procedure. Women aged 50 to 74 should have a mammogram every two years, although some medical professionals recommend starting earlier if risk factors are present.

- **Cervical Cancer**: Pap smears, combined with HPV testing, have dramatically reduced the rate of cervical cancer by catching precancerous lesions early. Women should begin Pap tests at age 21 and continue every three or five years; HPV tests start at age 30.

- **Colorectal Cancer**: Colonoscopies are vital for detecting colorectal cancer early and preventing it by removing precancerous polyps. Regular screenings should start at age 45 for most individuals. The procedure, although slightly uncomfortable, can be lifesaving.

- **Lung Cancer**: For those at high risk, particularly long-term heavy smokers, low-dose CT scans may detect lung cancer early when it is most treatable. Discuss with your healthcare provider if you are over 50 and have a history of smoking.

- **Skin Cancer**: Self-exams as well as regular skin checks by a healthcare professional are crucial for spotting early signs of skin cancer. Pay attention to any changes in moles, spots, or skin texture, and take photos to track changes. Dermatologists recommend routine checks, particularly for those at higher risk due to sun exposure or family history.

- **Prostate Cancer**: PSA blood tests and digital rectal exams are recommended for men over 50 or younger men with a family history of prostate cancer. Symptoms like changes in urination or blood in the urine should not be ignored. Discuss the pros and cons of screening with your doctor to make an informed decision.

- **Ovarian Cancer**: There are currently no effective broad screening tests for ovarian cancer in women without symptoms and who are at average risk. Doctors may, however, recommend transvaginal ultrasounds and CA-125 blood tests as part of a monitoring strategy for women with a high risk due to family history or women who have specific genetic markers.

- **Pancreatic Cancer**: Screening for pancreatic cancer is generally recommended only for individuals at high risk due to family history or genetic factors. Tests may include imaging studies such as MRI, CT scans, and endoscopic ultrasounds to monitor changes in the pancreas.

By proactively scheduling regular cancer screenings, you can catch potential issues before they become life-threatening and give yourself the best possible chances for a long, healthy life.

Similarly, screenings for high blood pressure, cholesterol levels, and diabetes play a pivotal role in identifying risk factors for heart disease and stroke, again enabling individuals and healthcare providers to intervene with lifestyle changes or medication before conditions worsen.

Lifestyle Changes You Can Make

The lifestyle choices we make daily are the foundation of preventative health. Nutrition, physical activity, weight management, and the avoidance of harmful habits contribute significantly to our life expectancy.

- **Nutrition:** A balanced diet rich in vegetables, whole grains, and lean proteins fuels the body with essential nutrients, supports immune function, and reduces the risk of chronic diseases
- **Physical Activity:** Regular exercise strengthens the cardiovascular system, boosts mental health, helps maintain a healthy weight, and reduces the risk of type 2 diabetes, heart disease, and certain cancers.
- **Weight Management:** Achieving and maintaining a healthy weight through balanced nutrition and regular physical activity can prevent the onset of obesity-related diseases.
- **Avoiding Harmful Habits:** Staying away from cigarettes and limiting alcohol consumption are critical to good health. Smoking is a leading cause of cancer and heart disease, and excessive alcohol intake can lead to liver disease, mental health problems, and an increased risk of accidents.

The approach to healthcare is evolving, moving toward more personalized and preventative strategies. This shift promises a future when healthcare is tailored to each individual's unique genetic makeup, lifestyle, and family history. Armed with knowledge and tools that empower you to make informed decisions, you will play an active role in your health journey.

Unlocking Your Health Blueprint

Some of the knowledge that will empower your greater participation in your healthcare will come from genomics, the study of your genes and their functions. This analysis will yield a blueprint of your body, insights into how your genetic makeup can influence your health, help in predicting the risk of certain diseases, and clues about how you might respond to certain medications, all of this leading to more personalized and more effective treatments.

- **Consider Genetic Testing:** If you're at risk for genetic conditions, genetic testing can be a powerful tool for developing preventative strategies. Testing is available for the BRCA1 and BRCA2 gene mutations that significantly increase the risk of breast and ovarian cancer. Similarly, sickle cell disease can be detected through genetic testing, helping those with a family history of the condition manage it early on. Familial hypercholesterolemia, a genetic condition that causes high cholesterol, can also be identified, allowing individuals to make critical lifestyle adjustments or begin treatment early. Talk to your healthcare provider to see if genetic testing is right for you.
- **Stay Informed & Talk to Your Family:** In addition to keeping up with advancements in genomics and disease prevention, know your family's health history. Family history often holds clues about inherited conditions, like heart disease or certain cancers, that may not be evident in genetic tests alone. Knowing this information can help you and your doctor design a personalized health plan to mitigate risks.

Consistent Checkups Are Key

Regular checkups do more than offer peace of mind; they can help catch health issues early. Routine visits for physical and mental health ensure that you're staying on top of any potential concerns before they become bigger problems.

- **Schedule Annual Checkups:** Schedule annual checkups: Don't wait for symptoms to appear. Regular visits to your primary care physician (PCP), dentist, and optometrist can help detect health issues before they escalate. Your PCP can monitor cholesterol and blood pressure, your dentist can keep track of your oral health, and your optometrist can detect early signs of conditions like glaucoma, cataracts, or even systemic diseases such as diabetes and high blood pressure. All this information from key healthcare professionals is vital for your overall well-being.

- **Monitor Your Mental Health:** Your mental health is as crucial as our physical health. Being open with your healthcare provider about your mental and emotional well-being during checkups will ensure a holistic approach to your care.

- **Be Involved in Decisions about Your Health:** Take an active role in your healthcare. As you thoroughly discuss treatment options with your provider, be sure you understand both the benefits and the risks, so that you can make informed decisions that align with your personal health goals.

- **Know Your Family Health History**
- As mentioned above, your family's health history is an invaluable tool that can help predict potential health risks you might face at some point. Knowing which conditions run in your family can guide your healthcare provider's recommendations about specific preventative measures.

- **Common Family Health Risks:** Conditions like early menopause, heart disease, diabetes, breast cancer, colon cancer, and even mental health conditions often have genetic components. It's essential to gather as much information as possible about these issues.

- **Gather Information:** Talk to relatives about their medical history, including the age at which they were diagnosed with specific conditions. Keep a record of any chronic diseases, early-onset conditions, or hereditary cancers.

- **Share with Your Healthcare Provider:** Provide this information to your doctors during checkups. A comprehensive family health history helps them tailor screening recommendations and preventative strategies specifically to you.

By staying informed and proactive, you can manage your health better and address potential risks before they become critical.

Simon Gets a Wake-Up Call

> Simon, a 45-year-old construction worker and dad, was always exhausted. He blamed long hours, ignoring 15 extra pounds and dizzy spells. At a free health fair, a nurse checked his blood sugar: 132 mg/dL, signaling prediabetes. Carlos, whose dad lost a leg to diabetes, felt shaken. A community clinic nurse helped him start small. He swapped soda for water, added beans and spinach to meals, and walked 20 minutes daily with his kids. Monthly clinic visits tracked his A1c. Six months later, Carlos lost 10 pounds, his blood sugar normalized, and he had energy to play soccer with his son. That health fair was more than a checkup…it was a lifeline.

Your Environment Matters

Where you live, work, and spend your time has a significant impact on your health and well-being. The air you breathe, the water you drink, and the spaces you inhabit all influence your physical and mental health. Whether you live in a bustling city or a rural area, environmental factors can either support or hinder your health. Clean air, safe drinking water, and access to nature can improve your well-being; pollution and overcrowding can lead to health issues.

You won't have control over every aspect of your environment, but you can take practical steps to both protect yourself and enhance your surroundings. If, for example, you live in a busy urban area with poor air quality, you can prioritize spending time in nature, seek indoor spaces with air purifiers, or advocate for cleaner energy solutions in your community. If water quality is a concern, using home filtration systems can help ensure you're drinking clean water.

Be mindful of your surroundings and then take steps to improve or mitigate the effects of environmental factors on your health.

What You Can Do to Improve Your Environment:

- **Improve Indoor Air Quality**: If outdoor air quality is poor, control the air quality in your home by keeping windows closed on high pollution days, using air purifiers, and not smoking indoors.
- **Spend Time in Nature**: Regular exposure to green spaces can reduce stress, elevate mood, and promote physical activity. If you live in a

crowded urban area, seek out local parks or plan weekend trips to more open, natural spaces.
- **Drink Clean Water**: Ensure the water you drink is safe by using filters if necessary. Staying hydrated with clean water is essential to good health.
- **Reduce Exposure to Pollutants**: Pay attention to local air quality reports and avoid outdoor activities when pollution levels are high. Consider using nontoxic cleaning products in your home to reduce your exposure to chemicals.

By making these small, manageable changes, you'll create a healthier environment for yourself and your family. You can take control of how your environment affects your health.

Air Quality and Respiratory Health

Air pollution is a harmful mixture of particulate matter, chemicals, and gases that directly impacts respiratory health. According to the World Health Organization, air pollution leads to approximately 7 million premature deaths annually, with respiratory conditions like asthma, chronic bronchitis, and lung cancer being major contributors. Children and the elderly are especially vulnerable: air pollutants can worsen asthma symptoms in children and contribute to the development of chronic obstructive pulmonary disease (COPD) in adults.

To minimize your exposure to unhealthy air, check a weather app or an air quality index to stay informed about local air quality. Limit outdoor activities on high-pollution days, and take precautions to protect your lungs, such as wearing a well-fitted N95 mask if you need to be outside or exercising indoors instead. When you're indoors, using air purifiers and keeping windows closed during peak pollution times can help maintain clean air. Proper ventilation is key as well — once outdoor air quality improves, briefly opening windows or using exhaust fans can help clear out indoor pollutants like cooking fumes or chemicals that build up when a home is sealed tightly against outdoor air.

Improving Indoor Air Quality: Consider bringing in spider plants or peace lilies that can help filter out toxins. If you live near a busy road, planting outdoor greenery as a barrier can help reduce the impact of outdoor pollutants entering your living space.

Tobacco Smoke and Vaping: If you smoke or vape, doing so outdoors is crucial to keeping others in your household healthy. Smoke and vape particles can linger indoors, affecting air quality and the health of children and pets.

Everyday Chemical Exposure: Daily exposure to chemicals in household cleaners, personal care products, and food packaging can accumulate, leading to health risks such as hormone disruption and cancer. The Environmental Working Group (EWG) reports that many everyday products contain chemicals linked to reproductive harm, developmental issues, and cancer. Use natural or homemade cleaning products and choose cosmetics free of harmful chemicals. Being mindful of product labels and opting for certified organic products can further minimize chemical exposure.

Additionally, reducing the use of plastics including hard plastics like Tupperware, plastic wraps, and plastic bags, especially for food storage can decrease exposure to endocrine-disrupting chemicals like BPA and phthalates. Instead, opt for safer alternatives like glass, stainless steel, or silicone containers for storing food and beverages.

Water Quality

Clean water is foundational to good health, and for most people in affluent nations like the US, drinking water is generally very safe. Occasional contamination can still occur, and contaminants like lead, mercury, and microorganisms can cause serious health issues, including neurological damage and gastrointestinal diseases. The Centers for Disease Control and Prevention (CDC) report that lead exposure can contribute to developmental issues in children and kidney problems in adults.

To ensure your water is safe, consider using water filters that target specific contaminants, and if you're unsure about local water quality, drink bottled water. When traveling, especially to regions where water safety is a concern, it's a good idea to boil water or use purification tablets.

Noise Pollution

Excessive noise from traffic, industrial activities, or urban development can significantly impact mental health, causing stress, sleep disturbances, and even cardiovascular issues. The World Health Organization (WHO) considers noise pollution a major environmental health risk, contributing to problems like heart disease, cognitive impairment in children, and disrupted sleep patterns.

To reduce your exposure to noise pollution, you can take some practical steps at home. Start by soundproofing your living spaces with heavy curtains or rugs that will help absorb sound. You can also use plants, both indoors and outside, to create a natural noise barrier. Hedges and plants like bamboo are excellent at reducing noise levels. Moving your sleeping space to the quietest room in the house or using a white noise machine can also help improve sleep quality.

Whenever you are able to spend time outdoors, choose quieter locations to relax. If you can't avoid a noisy environment, consider wearing earplugs.

The Impact of Climate Change on Health

Climate change, including heatwaves and extreme weather events, exacerbates health risks, including the spread of infectious diseases. The WHO estimates that between 2030 and 2050, climate change is expected to cause approximately 250,000 additional deaths per year from malnutrition, malaria, diarrhea, and heat stress. To combat these risks, we can all support and engage in sustainability practices, such as reducing carbon emissions and conserving water. Additionally, we can advocate for policies that address climate change and its impact on health. Each of us can also prepare for extreme weather events by staying informed and having emergency plans in place. Promoting renewable energy sources and supporting reforestation projects can also mitigate the health impacts of climate change.

Green Spaces and Physical Health

Spending time in green spaces is essential for your physical and mental well-being. The WHO highlights that access to parks, gardens, and nature not only reduces stress and boosts mental health but also encourages physical activity, which is vital for overall health. Whether you go on a walk in the park during your lunch break, take a longer weekend hike, or simply relax in a garden, prioritizing time outdoors can have significant health benefits.

So make it a habit to seek out green spaces regularly. If your area lacks greenery, you might get involved in local community efforts that support urban projects like planting trees, creating rooftop gardens, or supporting community gardens.

These spaces not only provide recreational areas but also improve air quality and foster a sense of community. By participating, you not only benefit your own health but also contribute to the creation of healthier urban environments for everyone.

Electromagnetic Fields (EMFs) and Health

With the increasing use of electronic devices, concern about the health effects of electromagnetic fields (EMFs) has grown. Research continues, but some studies suggest that prolonged exposure to high levels of EMFs may increase the risk of cancer and other health issues. Radiofrequency electromagnetic fields are possibly carcinogenic. Minimizing exposure by using wired connections when possible, limiting the use of devices, especially before bedtime, and following guidelines for safe EMF levels can help reduce potential risks. Using speakerphone or wired headsets and avoiding the prolonged use of laptops on the lap can also mitigate exposure.

Digital Health Tools

In the age of technology, preventative health has been revolutionized by the rise of digital health tools and technologies. So although it's important to limit screen time and stay mindful of your tech habits, these innovative resources offer incredible ways for you to take control of your health. From apps that log daily food intake and track physical activity to wearable devices that monitor vital signs like heart rate, blood pressure, and even blood sugar levels, technology now provides real-time insights into your health.

You probably already have access to tools like these on your smartphone or smartwatch, so why not take a look today to see how your tech can support your health goals? Dietary apps can help you track what you eat and drink, providing valuable insights into your nutrition. Fitness trackers keep you motivated by setting goals, tracking your progress, and offering challenges. If you struggle with sleep, choose from among the apps that analyze your sleep cycles and suggest ways to improve your rest and recovery.

Wearable technologies like smartwatches can continuously monitor all that's going on in and with your body, giving you immediate feedback that could alert you to potential health issues early on. These tools enable you to be proactive, catching small health concerns before they become bigger problems. So, make the most of the technology at your fingertips to stay on track with your health goals!

Some common sense, basic medical information, knowledge of your family tree, wise choices about eating and exercising—these steps and others can help you build a healthier tomorrow today!

10 Ways to Protect Your Health: The Power of Prevention

1. Schedule Regular Checkups

Don't wait until you feel sick to see a doctor. Annual health screenings and routine checkups can catch diseases early when they're most treatable.

What to check:

- Blood pressure (under 120/80 mmHg)
- Cholesterol levels (LDL under 100 mg/dL)
- Blood sugar levels (fasting glucose under 100 mg/dL)
- Cancer screenings (mammograms, colonoscopies, skin checks)

2. Stay Up-to-Date with Vaccinations

Vaccines are one of the most powerful tools for preventing disease. Ensure you are up to date on these:

- Flu shot (yearly)
- Tdap booster (every 10 years for tetanus, diphtheria, and pertussis)
- Shingles vaccine (age 50 and older)
- Pneumonia vaccine (age 65 and older)

3. Eat Like Your Life Depends on It

A diet high in processed foods, sugar, and unhealthy fats increases the risk of diabetes, heart disease, and cancer.

4. Move Every Day

Exercise reduces the risk of nearly every chronic disease and keeps your body and mind sharp. You don't need to live in the gym. Just find activities you enjoy and do them.

Best exercises for longevity:

- Walking (30 minutes, five times per week)
- Strength training (twice per week)
- Swimming or cycling (great for joint health)
- Dancing (fun, social, and effective)

5. Maintain a Healthy Weight

Carrying extra weight, especially around the midsection, increases the risk of diabetes, heart disease, and joint pain. Instead of obsessing over the scale, focus on:

- Healthy eating habits
- Building muscle (not just losing weight)
- Moving daily

6. Quit Smoking & Cut Back on Alcohol

Smoking and excessive alcohol speed up aging, increase cancer risk, and damage nearly every organ in the body.

7. Prioritize Mental Health

Mental health is just as important as physical health. Unchecked stress leads to inflammation, poor sleep, and disease. Manage it by:

- Practicing meditation or deep breathing
- Taking walks outside
- Journaling about your thoughts and worries
- Seeking therapy or talking to a friend

8. Sleep As If It Were Your Job

Poor sleep is linked to heart disease, weight gain, and cognitive decline. Prioritize 7 to 9 hours of quality sleep every night by:

- Setting a regular bedtime
- Avoiding screens an hour before bed
- Keeping your room dark and cool

9. Stay Informed

Knowledge is power, and knowing your personal risk factors helps you make smarter choices. Stay up-to-date on the following:

- The latest research on nutrition, fitness, and disease prevention
- Family history: know your genetic risks
- Preventative screenings for heart disease, diabetes, and cancer

10. Build a Strong Support System: Health Is a Team Sport

You are more likely to stay healthy when you're surrounded by upbeat and like-minded people. Your social circle affects your habits more than you realize.

- Find accountability partners.
- Share healthy meals with friends and family.
- Join a workout group or participate in a community event.

Your Action Plan for Prevention

Good health doesn't happen by accident. The strongest bodies and sharpest minds are built through daily choices. So come up with a plan for prevention and get ahead of health problems before they start.

1. Your Health Snapshot: Where Are You Right Now?

Take a moment to assess where you stand today before considering changes.

When was your last complete physical checkup? Did you address mental health too?

Do you know your latest health numbers?

- ☐ Blood Pressure: _____
- ☐ Cholesterol (LDL & HDL levels): _____
- ☐ Fasting Blood Sugar: _____

What screening tests are overdue?

- ☐ Annual physical
- ☐ Blood pressure, cholesterol, and/or glucose test
- ☐ Cancer screening (mammogram, colonoscopy, skin check)
- ☐ Bone density scan (if over 50 or at risk for osteoporosis)

2. Upgrade Your Disease Defense: Are Your Vaccines Current?

Vaccinations are one of the simplest ways to protect your future self.

Which of these do you need to schedule?

- ☐ Flu shot (yearly)
- ☐ Tdap booster (every 10 years)

- [ ] Shingles vaccine (age 50+)
- [ ] Pneumonia vaccine (age 65+)

3. Food as Medicine: Revamp Your Diet

Every bite you take is either fueling health or feeding disease.

What is one processed or unhealthy food you will cut back on this week?

What is one nutrient-dense food you will add more of?

- [ ] If cutting out soda feels impossible, switch to sparkling water.
- [ ] If vegetables are an afterthought, start adding a handful of greens to one meal per day.

4. Movement Is Medicine: Find What Works for You

Your body was built to move, and movement is actually one of the most powerful ways to fight disease.

Which activities do you enjoy?

- [ ] Walking (30 minutes, five times per week)
- [ ] Strength training (twice per week)
- [ ] Swimming or cycling (gentle on joints)
- [ ] Dancing, hiking, or active hobbies

What's one small way you can move more this week?

Example: Take the stairs instead of the elevator or stretch for five minutes in the morning.

5. Body Composition: Shift the Focus from Weight to Strength

Forget the scale. True health is about muscle, energy, and mobility.

What's one muscle, energy, or mobility goal you want to work toward?

Example: Feel stronger, have more endurance, fit into a favorite outfit.

What's one small change in your diet you will make this week?

Example: Swap one processed snack for protein or fiber-rich food.

6. Cut the Harm, Strengthen Your Body

Smoking, excessive alcohol, and poor sleep weaken your immune system and speed up aging.

Which harmful habit do you want to cut back on?

What is one small step you will take?

- ☐ Skip alcohol on weekdays.
- ☐ Reduce smoking by one cigarette per day.
- ☐ Set a caffeine cut-off time.

7. Protect Your Mental Health as Well as Your Physical Health

Your brain and body are deeply connected: unchecked stress can lead to inflammation, weight gain, and chronic disease.

What's your number one source of stress right now?

Which of these will you commit to doing for stress relief?

- ☐ Five minutes of deep breathing
- ☐ Journaling for mental clarity

- [ ] Spending more time outside

- [ ] Scheduling therapy or a mental health check-in

8. The Sleep Audit: Are You Getting Enough?

Poor sleep is linked to heart disease, weight gain, and cognitive decline.

On average, how many hours of sleep are you currently getting every night?

What's one change you will make to improve your sleep quality?

- [ ] Set a consistent bedtime.

- [ ] Avoid screens an hour before bed.

- [ ] Keep your room cool and dark.

9. Stay Informed: Build Health Knowledge That Serves You

The more you know, the better choices you can make.

What's one health topic you want to know more about or understand better?

Where will you get your information?

- [ ] Read a book or article.

- [ ] Listen to a health podcast.

- [ ] Ask my doctor at my next appointment.

10. Build a Health-Focused Social Circle

Each one of us is the average of the five people we spend the most time with.

Who in your life supports your health goals?

What will you do to engage with a health-minded community?

☐ Join a walking or fitness group.

☐ Cook healthy meals with the family.

☐ Find an accountability partner.

Taking the First Steps

Remember, the journey of preventative health doesn't require perfection; it's about making more health-conscious choices more often. Each step, no matter how small, is a victory. Start with one or two changes and build from there. Over time, these choices become habits, and these habits become your foundation for a healthier life.

You have the power to improve your health. By adopting preventative health measures, you're not just avoiding disease; you're also choosing to live your life to its full potential. So take that first step today, for yourself and for those who love you. Your future self will thank you.

CHAPTER 8

HEALTH FOR ALL WOMEN:

ADDRESSING OUR UNIQUE NEEDS AND MAINTAINING LONG-TERM WELLNESS

BY RANI RAMASWAMY, MD

A ballet instructor who had dedicated her life to fitness and health, Sarah was passionate about inspiring her students in the small town where she'd opened her own dance studio.

When she was diagnosed with advanced breast cancer, it sent shockwaves through her family and the entire community. Sarah, who had always been the embodiment of strength, suddenly faced a grueling treatment plan that tested her body and her spirit.

Despite the challenges, Sarah continued to teach, adjusting her movements as her strength faded but never losing the poise and grace that her students admired. Her studio became a place of quiet resilience: she remained dedicated to her craft even as cancer altered the rhythm of her life.

As her illness progressed, Sarah focused on spending meaningful time with her loved ones. Although her body grew weaker, her spirit remained vibrant, and her family cherished every moment they had with her. Sarah passed away peacefully, leaving behind a community deeply affected by her loss. Her death raised questions that resonate with many: How could someone who led such a healthy, active life succumb to cancer?

This story highlights a critical truth about women's health: although essential, physical fitness and a healthy lifestyle are not always enough to shield us from disease. We women face unique health risks due to the biological, hormonal, and genetic factors that can make us more susceptible to certain conditions like breast cancer, heart disease, and autoimmune disorders. Understanding these risks and focusing on preventative care, regular screenings, and early intervention can make all the difference in maintaining long-term wellness. This chapter will dive deeper into the complexities of women's health, emphasizing the importance of personalized care and the proactive steps every woman can take to protect her well-being.

***

Women's health is an essential and distinct field within healthcare, meriting focused attention due to the unique biological and social factors that influence women's health outcomes. It's crucial to focus specifically on women's health and how various factors impact your overall well-being because hormones like estrogen and progesterone play pivotal roles in shaping your health, influencing everything from reproductive functions to cardiovascular health and bone density. Estrogen not only regulates your menstrual cycle and affects reproductive health but also influences cholesterol metabolism, which can impact the risk of heart disease risk. Understanding your hormones and how they interact within your body can help you address specific health concerns such as menstrual irregularities, pregnancy, menopause, and conditions like polycystic ovary syndrome (PCOS) and endometriosis.

Research shows that hormonal changes also significantly affect mental health. For instance, fluctuating hormones during the menstrual cycle can lead to premenstrual syndrome (PMS) and its more severe form, premenstrual dysphoric disorder (PMDD), affecting a substantial percentage of women with symptoms severe enough to disrupt daily functioning. Moreover, during menopause, the sharp decline in estrogen levels is associated with an increased risk of osteoporosis and cardiovascular disease. Approximately 1 in 3 women over the age of 50 experience osteoporotic fractures, and heart disease becomes the leading cause of death in women post-menopause. People tend to think that heart disease is more prevalent in men, but the statistics show otherwise. Again, heart disease poses a serious risk for women, especially after menopause. Understanding this risk is crucial to women who want to protect their cardiovascular health as they age.

The Gender Disparity

Women face significant disparities in healthcare access and treatment often due to socioeconomic factors, cultural norms, and gender biases within medical research. A global study published in the British medical journal *The Lancet*, for instance, found that women are less likely to receive timely diagnoses and appropriate treatments for cardiovascular disease compared to men even though that disease is the leading cause of death for both genders. Additionally, only about 30% of participants in clinical trials for heart-related medications and treatments are women despite women comprising nearly half of the population. This gap in research and healthcare leaves women at a disadvantage when it comes to receiving care.

Women are often primary caregivers for family members, which can negatively impact their health because of the time-consuming and stressful demands of that role, leaving us with less time for personal healthcare. Studies suggest that the challenges of balancing work and family life contribute to the higher prevalence of autoimmune diseases in women because chronic stress can exacerbate these conditions. In addition, societal expectations and roles can lead to health issues. In some cultures, for example, women are expected to prioritize caregiving over self-care, and those expectations can keep women from receiving immediate medical attention.

Research also shows that some social groups are less likely to exercise than others. A study conducted by Harvard University revealed that women, particularly those from lower socioeconomic backgrounds, are 30% less likely to engage in regular physical activity than men are. This disparity further impacts women's health, contributing to the risk of obesity, cardiovascular disease, and other chronic conditions.

Moreover, societal norms can also hinder women from seeking help for conditions related to reproductive and sexual health. In some conservative communities, for instance, discussing issues like menstruation or sexual health may still be stigmatized, and late diagnoses of conditions such as polycystic ovary syndrome (PCOS) or cervical cancer may result. These barriers prevent women from receiving timely and appropriate care, exacerbating their health issues.

Your Reproductive System

Although many women are familiar with the basic functions of the reproductive system, understanding the nuances of how these processes affect our overall health is key. Menstrual health, fertility, and the transitions into perimenopause and menopause all have a significant impact on a woman's physical and emotional well-being. The hormonal shifts that accompany these stages can affect cardiovascular health, bone density, and mental well-being as well as general reproductive health. Therefore, focusing on how each phase of the reproductive cycle interconnects with the rest of your body is critical to addressing women's health holistically.

When we consider the broader implications of reproductive health and how it affects a woman's body overall, we can better understand the importance of prioritizing regular healthcare checkups. We need to be aware of any signs that may indicate underlying conditions, such as polycystic ovary syndrome (PCOS), endometriosis, or issues with fertility.

Priya's PCOS Journey

> Priya, a 30-year-old teacher, felt defeated by irregular periods, weight gain, and acne. A telehealth visit diagnosed PCOS, a turning point. Priya swapped chips for quinoa and leafy greens, danced to music for 30 minutes daily, and journaled to ease stress. Her doctor checked in monthly via video calls. Four months later, Priya lost 8 pounds, her periods returned, and her skin cleared. She looked in the mirror and smiled, feeling in control for the first time in years.

Hormonal Fluctuations

Hormones play a crucial role in regulating many processes in the female body. Estrogen and progesterone not only regulate the menstrual cycle but also influence various other body systems, including the cardiovascular and the skeletal systems. Hormonal changes are especially significant during key life phases such as pregnancy, breastfeeding, and menopause. However, it's important to note that symptoms associated with menopause, such as hot flashes, mood swings, and increased risk of osteoporosis, can actually begin in the years leading up to menopause, years known as perimenopause.

Starting in their early forties and even earlier for some women, perimenopause is marked by fluctuating hormone levels that can lead to symptoms long before periods stop entirely. These changes are often misunderstood because many women believe that certain symptoms they experience only begin after menopause. Also less well-known is the broader impact hormonal fluctuations can have on the body, such as affecting sleep quality, skin health, and even cognitive function. Recognizing these shifts before the onset of menopause is crucial for managing symptoms and protecting long-term health.

- **Cardiovascular System:** Estrogen helps maintain the flexibility of the arteries, allowing them to easily accommodate blood flow. As estrogen levels drop during menopause, the risk of developing cardiovascular diseases increases due to stiffer arteries and a potential rise in cholesterol levels.
- **Bone Health:** Estrogen is vital to bone growth and maintenance. It helps balance the remodeling process during which old bone tissue is replaced by new bone tissue. Reduced estrogen levels during menopause accelerate bone loss, increasing the risk of osteoporosis.
- **Metabolic Changes:** Women experience unique metabolic changes, especially during pregnancy (gestational diabetes) and menopause (increased risk of weight gain and metabolic syndrome). These changes can affect their long-term metabolic health, influencing risks for conditions like type 2 diabetes and cardiovascular diseases.
- **Mental Health:** Hormonal fluctuations can also impact mental health. Changes in estrogen and progesterone levels can affect neurotransmitter systems in the brain, influencing mood, emotional well-being, and the prevalence of anxiety and depression.

Preventative Health

Understanding how your body changes over time is key to taking control of your health. Regular screenings such as mammograms for breast cancer, Pap smears for cervical cancer, and bone density tests for osteoporosis are essential tools for catching potential issues early. While these tests are widely available, it's important to talk to your healthcare provider to determine when you should start regularly taking each one. Recommendations may vary depending on your personal and family health history.

In addition to these regular periodic screenings, you can take other proactive steps to stay ahead of health concerns. Maintaining a balanced diet rich in calcium and Vitamin D can support your bone health, and regular exercise helps you strengthen your cardiovascular system and manage your weight. Monitoring your hormonal changes whether by tracking your menstrual cycle or being aware of perimenopausal symptoms can help you better understand what's going on in your body and address any issues early. Preventative health is about making informed, everyday choices that can protect your well-being now and in the future.

Reproductive Health

Encompassing everything from menstruation to menopause, reproductive health is intertwined with a woman's overall well-being whether she chooses to have children or not. So what can you do to look after your reproductive health?

- Understand menstruation not just as a physical health process but also as an indicator of overall health. Issues such as heavy bleeding, severe pain, or irregular cycles can be signs of underlying health problems that require medical attention.
- Contraception offers women control over their reproductive planning, but choosing the right method can be daunting. Options range from hormonal pills to long-acting contraceptives like IUDs. Each method has its benefits and its side effects, and what works best will depend on the individual's health, personal needs, and lifestyle.
- Pregnancy necessitates increased healthcare monitoring to ensure the health of both the mother and the developing fetus. Common concerns during pregnancy include gestational diabetes, preeclampsia,

and the baby's health. Regular prenatal care is crucial to effectively managing these risks. It's also important to understand that pregnancy can have long-term effects on a woman's health. Conditions like gestational diabetes can increase the risk of developing type 2 diabetes later in life, and preeclampsia may raise the risk of cardiovascular disease. Additionally, pregnancy-related changes to the body, such as pelvic floor issues or postpartum depression, may require ongoing care and attention even after childbirth. Getting regular checkups and addressing any lingering health concerns post-pregnancy is essential to safeguarding a woman's long-term well-being.

- Menopause marks the end of a woman's reproductive years and can bring significant hormonal changes that affect both physical and mental health. Symptoms like broken sleep, mood swings, changes to skin and hair, and vaginal discomfort can be challenging. These symptoms can often be managed through lifestyle changes such as regular exercise, a balanced diet, and stress management techniques. For some women and depending on her individual risk factors and health considerations hormone replacement therapy (HRT) may be a suitable option to relieve more severe symptoms. It's important to consult with a healthcare provider to explore the best approach for managing menopause.

Chronic Conditions

Knowing about the chronic conditions more common in women can help you stay alert to any symptoms. If you have any concerns, talk to your doctor as soon as possible. Early diagnosis and intervention are often key to more effective management and better outcomes.

- **Autoimmune Diseases**: Conditions like lupus and rheumatoid arthritis are significantly more common in women than men. These diseases cause your immune system to attack your body's own tissues, leading to inflammation and damage. Symptoms can vary widely but often include fatigue, joint pain, and skin rashes. If you notice any of these signs, seek medical advice promptly. Again, early diagnosis and treatment can help doctors effectively manage these conditions.
- **Osteoporosis**: Women are more prone to osteoporosis, particularly post-menopause, when lower estrogen levels accelerate bone density

loss. To reduce your risk, consider preventative measures such as hormone replacement therapy (HRT). Growing evidence suggests it helps protect bone health. Also be sure you're getting enough calcium and Vitamin D and engage in regular weight-bearing exercise like walking, jogging, or strength training. In addition, lifestyle modifications like not smoking and limiting alcohol consumption can help maintain strong bones.

- **Cancer**: Breast and ovarian cancers are significant health concerns for women. Regular mammograms can detect breast cancer early when it's most treatable, but it's equally important to learn how you yourself can check for changes in your breasts. Make a habit of regularly checking for any lumps or unusual changes when you're in the shower or in front of a mirror. Ovarian cancer is more challenging to detect early, so it's crucial to be aware of symptoms like bloating, pelvic pain, or frequent urination. If you have a family history of these cancers, discuss genetic testing and preventative strategies with your healthcare provider so you can take proactive steps.

- **Go to Screening Appointments**

    Whenever it's time to go for a regular screening, *go!* These checkups and tests are vital for catching diseases early, often before symptoms even appear, and that's when those diseases are most treatable. Some women, especially younger ones, may delay or avoid mammograms and Pap smears, sometimes due to fear or discomfort, but these tests can save your life. Any discomfort is minimal compared to the benefits. So make your health a priority.

    To help you do just that, here are three critical screenings you should never skip:

- **Pap Smears for Cervical Cancer**: If you're between the ages of 21 and 65, make sure you're getting regular Pap smears. This test collects cells from your cervix to check for any abnormalities that might develop into cervical cancer. It's quick, typically only slightly uncomfortable, and able to detect changes early on when treatment is most effective. If you're nervous about the procedure, talk to your doctor—and keep in mind that this test is about protecting your health. Pap smears are typically recommended every three years or, when combined with HPV testing, every five years.

- **Mammograms for Breast Cancer**: Most women begin getting regular mammograms at age 40, but women with a family history will start earlier. These X-rays can detect breast cancer even before you can feel a lump. Annual or biennial screenings are the norm with the frequency depending on your age and risk factors. Early detection of breast cancer thanks to mammograms drastically improves the chances of successful treatment. Also, don't forget to regularly perform self-checks at home. Make it a habit to feel for any unusual changes when you're in the shower or in front of a mirror. You know your body best, so trust your instincts and consult a doctor if something feels off.
- **Bone Density Tests for Osteoporosis**: Women are at greater risk of osteoporosis, especially after menopause, than men are. Therefore bone density tests are recommended for all women at age 65 and for younger women who are at high risk. This category includes women with a family history of osteoporosis, those who are thin or have low body weight, smokers, or women who used steroids for a long time. The early diagnosis made possible by these tests can help you take steps—starting medication and/or making lifestyle changes—to strengthen your bones and prevent fractures.

By staying current with these screenings, you're actively taking control of your health. Understandably, the possibility of cancer or osteoporosis may feel overwhelming and scary, but taking these proactive steps and getting these screenings will give you the best possible chance to detect problems early and keep yourself healthy.

Health at Any Age

Understanding how your health needs change with age is key to maintaining long-term wellness. Each decade of life brings new challenges and shifts in your body, and recognizing these changes can help you stay proactive about your health. Here are some things to keep in mind whatever decade of life you are in:

In Your 20s:

- **Hormonal Balance:** Depending on your body, you may notice changes in your menstrual cycle: periods might become more regular or stay irregular. It's also common for young women to start using contraception during this decade, and that can impact your hormones. If you're experiencing irregular periods or you have other menstrual concerns, be sure to discuss them with your healthcare provider.

- **Sexual and Mental Health:** The decisions you make now about sexual health like practicing safe sex and getting regular STI screenings are important for your overall well-being. Also, managing stress in healthy ways is essential during this busy decade of self-discovery, relationships, and career-building. Pay attention to your mental health and don't hesitate to seek support if you feel overwhelmed.

- **Work-Life Balance:** It's common to feel stretched thin between your work, your social life, and your need for personal time. Prioritize sleep, manage stress, and carve out time for physical activity whether you do yoga, a sport, or regular stretching. These habits will benefit you for years to come.

In Your 30s:

- **Fertility and Pregnancy:** Many women have their first child in their 30s. Fertility naturally declines, particularly after age 35, so if you'd like to have children, be sure to talk openly with your doctor about fertility and reproductive health. That said, women are increasingly having healthy pregnancies later in life.

- **Chronic Conditions:** Thyroid disorders, autoimmune diseases, and other chronic conditions often arise in this decade, so be aware of any unusual fatigue or changes in weight. Early detection and treatment are key to managing these conditions.

- **Finding Time for You:** Between work, family, and life responsibilities, it's easy to let self-care slip. This decade is crucial for establishing and maintaining good habits regarding fitness, stretching, and stress relief. Try to incorporate regular movement into your day and make time for activities that relax and restore you.

In Your 40s:

- **Perimenopause:** Hormonal changes may begin as you approach menopause. You might notice symptoms such as feeling low, broken sleep, or increased anxiety all of which can be connected to hormonal shifts. Many women are familiar with hot flashes, but these three more subtle symptoms are less often recognized as hormonal. Speak with your doctor if you're feeling low, struggling to sleep, or experiencing anxiety because certain treatments and lifestyle adjustments can help.

- **Breast Health:** Begin regular mammograms at age 40 to monitor breast health. The risk of breast cancer increases as you age, so early detection is essential.

- **Strength and Balance:** If you aren't already doing weight-bearing exercises and strength training, activities that can help maintain muscle mass and bone density, start now. Also make time for balance exercises, like yoga, to help prevent falls and maintain overall stability.

In Your 50s and Beyond:

- **Menopause:** As estrogen levels decrease, the risk of conditions like osteoporosis and cardiovascular disease increases. Talk to your doctor about hormone replacement therapy (HRT) to help manage symptoms like hot flashes, mood swings, and vaginal discomfort. HRT also provides some protection for bone and heart health. Remember, it's never too late to start making healthy changes!

- **Screenings:** Regular screenings are even more important during this decade. Get a mammogram every one to two years, and if you haven't already, have a baseline bone density test to check for osteoporosis. Colonoscopies should begin at age 50 to screen for colon cancer. Watch for changes in bowel habits and discuss any irregularities or blood in your stool with your doctor.

- **Diet and Alcohol:** Post-menopause, your cholesterol levels are likely to rise, so it's crucial to closely monitor your cardiovascular health. Eating a heart-healthy diet with plenty of fruits, vegetables, and whole grains and limiting alcohol to under eight units a week can help you stay healthy and strong.

By recognizing the unique health needs of each decade, you can proactively maintain your well-being and enjoy a vibrant, healthy life now and for years to come.

Look After Yourself at Any Age

Taking a proactive approach to wellness allows you to effectively manage your health in every decade of life. When you do so, you not only improve your quality of life today but you also prevent the development of more serious health issues later on.

- **Diet:** A balanced diet is key to feeling your best for as long as possible. Specifically, your diet should be rich in calcium for bone health, fiber for digestion, lean proteins for muscle maintenance, and plenty of vegetables to provide essential vitamins and nutrients. Eating well supports everything from energy level to immune function and helps protect against chronic diseases like heart disease, diabetes, and osteoporosis.
- **Exercise:** Regular physical activity is crucial for maintaining your strength, balance, and flexibility as you age. Consistent exercising also supports metabolic and cardiovascular health, keeps your muscles and joints strong, and reduces the risk of falls and fractures. Whether you choose brisk walking, swimming, or strength training, aim for at least 30 minutes of exercise most days to enhance both your physical and mental well-being.
- **Stress Management:** Chronic stress can lead to imbalances in your hormones and negatively impact your overall health. Manage stress through mindfulness techniques, yoga, meditation, or other activities that promote relaxation. Ensuring you get adequate sleep is also vital for recovery from the demands of everyday life.
- **Regular Screenings:** Make regular health screenings, like Pap smears, HPV vaccinations, mammograms, and breast self-exams, a part of your routine. Self-checks are just as important as doctor visits. Regularly checking your breasts and being aware of any changes in your body can lead to early detection of health issues. Consult your healthcare provider to discuss the recommended frequency of these screenings based on your age and health history.

Sexual Health

Our sexual health is an essential aspect of our overall well-being. It often doesn't receive the attention it deserves even though addressing and understanding sexual health can lead to improved physical, emotional, and mental health.

Sexual health includes the freedom to enjoy and the ability to control your sexual and reproductive choices without fear, discrimination, or shame. Access to accurate information as well as to safe, effective, and affordable contraception also contributes to sexual health. Primarily, though, sexual health is the ability to experience sexual pleasure, satisfaction, and intimacy when desired, the result being a balanced and fulfilling life.

By prioritizing sexual health, you empower yourself to make informed decisions, improve your quality of life, and nurture both your physical and emotional well-being.

Women's sexual health is influenced by a complex interplay of hormonal, physical, and psychological factors. Key hormones such as estrogen and progesterone significantly impact libido, vaginal health, and menstrual cycles, which in turn affect sexual function and satisfaction.

- **Estrogen** helps maintain vaginal tissue moisture and elasticity and plays a role in increasing blood flow to the pelvic region, enhancing sexual arousal.

- **Progesterone** can have varying effects on libido. Some women experience increased sexual desire while others may sense a decline especially during the luteal phase of the menstrual cycle.

- **Supporting Your Sexual Health**
  The World Health Organization highlights that sexual health issues are among the top five health concerns for women aged 15 to 44. In fact, research shows that only about 60% of women in the US are satisfied with their sexual experiences. So what can you do to enhance and support your sexual well-being?

- **Vaginal Dryness:** Vaginal dryness, which is often linked to menopause due to decreased estrogen levels, can make sexual activity uncomfortable and even painful. It affects between 17% and 50% of women post-menopause. In addition to lubricants and moisturizers, topical estrogen (available in creams or inserts) can be an effective solution and is particularly helpful for women who may not want to use full transdermal hormone replacement therapy (HRT).

- **Decreased Libido:** Several factors can contribute to a decrease in sexual desire, including hormonal changes, stress, fatigue, psychological issues, and relationship difficulties. Studies show that about 32% of women experience low sexual desire. Addressing issues like anxiety and depression through therapy or medication can help restore sexual health. Additionally, regular exercise not only boosts overall stamina but can also improve body image and increase blood flow, which may enhance libido.

- **Sexually Transmitted Infections (STIs):** Women are biologically more vulnerable to STIs than men, and these STIs can lead to serious consequences, including infertility. HPV, chlamydia, and gonorrhea are particularly common among young women aged 15 to 24. According to the American Sexual Health Association, half of all sexually active individuals will contract an STI by age 25. Although annual screenings for STIs are more common in the US than other places, it's each woman's responsibility to stay vigilant about sexual health even if they're asymptomatic. Regular Pap smears and HPV vaccinations are essential preventative measures against cervical cancer and genital warts.

- **Diet:** A balanced diet rich in fruits, vegetables, and whole grains supports overall health and plays a significant role in regulating the hormones that can affect sexual function. Eating well not only improves your energy level but also helps maintain a healthy libido.

By understanding and proactively addressing your sexual health, you can improve your physical and emotional well-being, helping you feel more empowered and fulfilled in your personal life.

Hormone Replacement Therapy

Commonly used to alleviate symptoms associated with hormonal imbalances or deficiencies, hormone replacement therapy (HRT) is often prescribed to women during perimenopause and menopause. Its primary goal is to restore hormone levels, particularly estrogen, and thereby relieve the physical and emotional challenges of menopause like hot flashes, mood swings, and sleep disturbances that arise due to declining estrogen levels. Additionally, HRT can provide the preventative benefits of reducing the risk of osteoporosis and cardiovascular disease, both of which can be influenced by hormonal changes.

HRT comes in various forms, including tablets, skin patches, gels, and implants that deliver estrogen directly into the bloodstream. For women who still have a uterus, progesterone is included to protect against the risk of the endometrial cancer that can develop from estrogen-only treatment. Progesterone is especially important for women in perimenopause who still have periods and deal with fluctuating hormones.

Up to 75% of women experience menopausal symptoms. About one-third describe their symptoms as severe and therefore having a significant impact on their quality of life, including their sleep, their mood, and their overall well-being. Starting HRT closer to the onset of menopause, within 10 years of the last period, has been associated with a reduced risk of coronary heart disease, lowering that risk by up to 30%. Research published in the *Journal of the American Heart Association* further emphasizes that early initiation of HRT not only alleviates menopausal symptoms but also reduces overall mortality and cardiovascular events. These encouraging results underscore the long-term health benefits of timely treatment. Still, it's important to discuss with your healthcare provider your individual risk factors and the potential benefits of HRT.

Benefits of HRT

1. **Relief from Menopausal Symptoms**: The primary benefit of HRT is relief from common symptoms of menopause like broken sleep, feeling low, night sweats, vaginal dryness, and decreased sex drive. HRT can also help with symptoms like hair thinning, brain fog, and joint aches, symptoms that are often overlooked yet can have a significantly negative impact on quality of life. By managing such symptoms, HRT can improve daily functioning and overall emotional well-being.
2. **Osteoporosis Prevention**: Estrogen plays a crucial role in maintaining bone density. That's why HRT can help prevent osteoporosis, a condition where bones become fragile due to hormonal changes. By supplying estrogen, HRT helps slow down bone loss, reducing the risk of fractures that often occur with age due to the loss of bone density during menopause.
3. **Improved Heart Health**: Early initiation of HRT, particularly within 10 years of menopause, can offer protection against heart disease by maintaining healthier blood vessels and reducing cholesterol levels. Research is ongoing, but many studies show that timely use of HRT

can support cardiovascular health. The benefit does vary depending on individual health profiles and the timing of the therapy.
4. **Potential Cognitive Benefits**: Emerging research suggests that HRT may help lower the risk of dementia particularly when therapy begins in the early stages of menopause. Women tend to experience higher rates of dementia than men, and hormonal fluctuation during menopause may be a contributing factor. By maintaining estrogen levels, HRT may offer some protective benefits for brain health, although research is still underway.

Raising the topic of HRT in a broader conversation about your health can prompt your doctor to address not only menopause symptoms but also long-term concerns like osteoporosis, heart disease, and potentially even cognitive decline. Always discuss your personal risk factors and benefits with your healthcare provider so you will be able to make an informed decision.

Risks and Considerations

Although HRT offers significant benefits, it isn't suitable for everyone, and its potential risks must be carefully weighed against its benefits:

1. **Increased Risk of Certain Cancers:** The risk of breast and ovarian cancer can increase with certain types of HRT, particularly when taken for long periods. The specific risk depends on the duration of the patient's hormone use and the type of hormones used. So talk to your doctor about HRT and the various products available for you to try. Also, some media reporting on HRT has been based on outdated research. Modern studies suggest that HRT risks vary, and your doctor can help you find a treatment plan tailored to you.
2. **Risk of Blood Clots and Stroke:** HRT especially in pill form can increase the risk of blood clots and stroke. The risk of blood clots is lower when the patient uses transdermal patches, gels, and sprays. Also important to know when you're evaluating your options is that HRT may offer protection against some cancers (colorectal cancer, for instance).
3. **Side Effects:** Some women on HRT experience side effects such as bloating, breast tenderness, nausea, and headaches. If you're dealing with side effects, talk to your doctor about adjusting your dosage or

trying a different formulation that works for you without the discomfort.

Ultimately, it's essential to have a thorough conversation with your healthcare provider as you consider the risks and the benefits of HRT in the context of your individual health history and symptoms.

Who Should Consider HRT

HRT is particularly recommended for women who:

- Experience moderate to severe menopausal symptoms that significantly impact their quality of life
- Have a family history of osteoporosis or are at high risk of bone fractures
- Entered menopause prematurely (before the age of 40)

Again, it's important to decide whether or not to start HRT in consultation with a healthcare provider. If you choose to start the treatment, the general guideline is to use the lowest effective dose for the shortest duration needed to manage the symptoms. Regular follow-ups are essential to assessing whether the treatment is working and to monitor for any potential risks.

Hormone replacement therapy can be a life-giving option for women suffering severely from the effects of menopause. They'll likely notice substantial improvements in both their daily life and, later, in their long-term health as well. Again, work closely with your healthcare provider and together carefully weigh the potential risks and benefits specific to your situation. You want your treatment plan to meet your personal health needs and align with your goals.

Prioritizing women's health means recognizing the unique challenges women face across their lifespan and taking proactive steps to address them because when women are empowered to care for their health, families and communities thrive too.

10 Ways to Optimize YOUR Health

1. Stay Ahead with Essential Health Screenings

Regular screenings can detect diseases early on when they are most treatable. Schedule these key checkups:

- Pap smear & HPV test (every 3 to 5 years or as recommended)
- Mammogram (every 1 to 2 years starting at age 40)
- Bone density scan (for postmenopausal women or those at risk for osteoporosis)
- Colonoscopy (starting at age 45)
- Thyroid function test (especially if experiencing fatigue, hair loss, or weight changes)

2. Prioritize Sleep to Balance Hormones and Protect Brain Health

Poor sleep affects hormonal balance, weight gain, and cognitive function. Women, especially during perimenopause and menopause, experience shifts in melatonin, cortisol, and estrogen levels that can make sleep difficult.

Improve sleep by:

- Sticking to a consistent bedtime
- Avoiding screens an hour before bed
- Keeping the room cool and dark
- Practicing relaxation techniques like deep breathing or magnesium supplements

3. Manage Stress to Protect Your Heart and Hormones

Chronic stress increases cortisol, leading to weight gain, anxiety, and an increased risk of heart disease. Furthermore, women especially those juggling careers, family, and caregiving often put themselves last, adding to the stress of their life circumstances.

Manage stress by:

- Practicing daily mindfulness or breathing exercises
- Doing gentle yoga or stretching
- Spending time in nature or engaging in hobbies

4. Hydrate for Skin, Digestion, and Cellular Health

Proper hydration helps flush toxins from your body, keep your skin glowing, regulate your digestion, and increase your energy levels. Women's hydration needs change with hormonal shifts, especially during perimenopause when estrogen drops and affects fluid retention.

- Aim to drink at least 8 glasses of water daily.
- Increase hydration by eating water-rich foods like cucumbers, watermelon, strawberries, oranges, celery, and lettuce, and by drinking herbal teas or infused water with fruits and herbs.
- Reduce caffeine and alcohol that dehydrate the body.

5. Optimize Nutrition and Adjust Supplements Wisely

Nutritional needs change with age, pregnancy, and menopause. Support your body by eating a nutrient-dense diet and using supplements when necessary.

The following are key nutrients for women's health:

- Calcium & Vitamin D (for strong bones and osteoporosis prevention)
- Magnesium (for muscle relaxation, sleep, and PMS relief)
- Omega-3 fatty acids (for brain function and a reduction of inflammation)
- Iron (for energy especially during menstruation)
- Collagen & protein (for skin elasticity and muscle maintenance)

6. Monitor and Protect Your Mental Health

Often due to hormonal fluctuations, societal pressures, and life transitions, women experience anxiety and depression at twice the rate that men do.

If you're feeling overwhelmed, don't just push through. Seek support.

- Therapy and counseling can help you navigate stress, anxiety, and major life changes.
- Exercise and meditation will boost serotonin and dopamine.
- Prioritizing social connections can improve your mental well-being.

7. Consider Hormone Therapy for Menopause Relief

Hormonal shifts during perimenopause and menopause can bring hot flashes, weight gain, brain fog, and joint pain. Hormone replacement therapy (HRT) can be an effective option for managing these symptoms and protecting heart and bone health.

HRT may help in the following ways:

- Reduce hot flashes and night sweats
- Prevent osteoporosis
- Protect brain function
- Improve mood and increase energy

HRT is not for everyone, so discuss both your personal risks and the potential benefits with a doctor.

8. Make Yourself a Priority—And Push Away the Guilt as You Do

Women often prioritize others at the expense of their own health. Even as you juggle work, family, and social obligations, it's essential that you carve out time to care for yourself. Doing so is critical to your well-being.

Nonnegotiable self-care includes:

- Regular movement (yoga, walking, resistance training)
- Time for hobbies (reading, art, gardening)
- Saying no to overcommitments

9. Stay Connected to People to Increase Longevity and Happiness

Strong social connections reduce stress, improve mental health, and even extend a person's life.

Here are some ways you can build and maintain connection:

- Join a women's health community online or in-person.
- Make friendship and socializing a priority.
- Seek support groups if you're navigating perimenopause, infertility, or chronic illness.

10. Educate Yourself as You Take Charge of Your Health

Stay informed about new research, treatments, and lifestyle practices.

- Read books and articles on nutrition, fitness, and hormone health.
- Stay up-to-date on health screenings and personal risk factors.
- Ask questions at doctor visits and advocate for yourself.

Your Action Plan: Take Control Today

1. Choose One Health Habit to Improve This Week

Small, consistent actions lead to lasting change. Identify the aspect of your health that most needs your attention right now:

☐ Sleep and stress management

☐ Balanced nutrition and hydration

☐ Physical activity and movement

☐ Hormonal health and menopause support

☐ Mental health and emotional well-being

Write down one specific action you'll take this week to improve your health:

2. Schedule Any Overdue Health Screenings

Prevention is the most powerful tool for long-term health. When was your last checkup?

☐ Pap smear & HPV test (every 3 to 5 years)

☐ Mammogram (every 1 to 2 years starting at age 40)

☐ Bone density scan (for postmenopausal women or those at risk for osteoporosis)

☐ Colonoscopy (starting at age 45)

☐ Thyroid function test (especially if you're experiencing fatigue, hair loss, or weight change)

3. Create a Long-Term Health Vision

Your health choices today shape the way you'll feel in the future. Take a moment to visualize yourself 5, 10, or 20 years from now.

How do you want to feel as the years ahead unfold?

- ☐ Energized, strong, and mentally sharp
- ☐ Free of chronic pain and disease
- ☐ Hormonally in balance and not experiencing mood swings
- ☐ Confident and comfortable in my body

What actions will help you achieve the goal you identified in the previous question?

- ☐ Prioritizing strength and mobility exercises
- ☐ Managing stress and improving mental resilience
- ☐ Making nutrition and hydration a priority
- ☐ Seeking medical care and staying current with recommended screenings

Write down one long-term health goal you want to work toward:

You Deserve to Prioritize Your Health

Women often take care of everyone else first, so having a health plan for yourself is absolutely necessary. When you take care of yourself, you have more energy and strength for the people and activities that matter most to you.

Start today. **Your future self will thank you.**

CHAPTER 9

HEALTH FOR ALL MEN:

RECOGNIZING THE BARRIERS THAT KEEP US FROM SEEKING HELP

Michael, a 58-year-old high school teacher beloved by many, was known for his ready laugh and great stories. His students adored him, and he was a well-respected figure in his community. However, behind his vibrant persona, Michael had been neglecting his health for years, brushing off symptoms that required attention.

He dismissed his frequent nighttime trips to the bathroom, difficulty starting to urinate, and the persistent, dull ache in his lower back as merely signs of aging. When his wife noticed these changes, she encouraged him to see a doctor, but fear and a busy schedule kept him from making that important appointment.

It wasn't until a close friend shared his own personal health scare that Michael realized the gravity of his symptoms and finally sought medical advice. A routine PSA test, a marker for prostate health, returned with elevated levels and alarmed Mchael and his wife. He got a referral and made an appointment for further tests. The results of those confirmed Michael's worst fear: he had advanced prostate cancer that had already spread to other parts of his body.

The diagnosis shook Michael, his wife, and their two children, who had always viewed him as the indestructible pillar of their family. Despite the prognosis, Michael faced his treatment with courage and strength. He underwent several therapies, hoping to slow the progression of the disease. He constantly thought about his children, worrying about how they would cope with his illness and the prospect of losing him.

After six months, when Michael's life came to a peaceful end, his passing left a void in the hearts of his family, friends, and students. Michael's story, particularly his delayed visit to the doctor, serves as a powerful reminder of the importance of early detection and proactive healthcare.

His is a story that reminds all of us that our health is everything and that we must listen to our bodies and take care of ourselves—before it's too late.

***

In today's fast-paced world, men's health often takes a back seat to the very real demands of daily life. But given society's expectations, lifestyle choices we've made, and the unique health challenges men face throughout life, we men need to make our physical and mental health a priority. This chapter shines a light on men's health, emphasizing the importance of addressing health issues through prevention, early detection, and effective treatment.

Understanding men's health is the first step, and it involves more than the descriptions of common ailments. Understanding our health is also about recognizing the barriers both external and internal that keep us from seeking help and/or adopting healthier habits. Statistically, men are less likely than women to visit the doctor for regular checkups, too often unintentionally allowing treatable conditions to progress to more serious stages. Sadly, this tendency impacts their quality of life as well as their longevity.

Clearly, the role of prevention cannot be overstated. Regular screenings and checkups are vital tools for detecting diseases early on when they're the most manageable. Coupled with lifestyle modifications, such as a balanced diet, regular physical activity, and stress management, prevention is a powerful strategy for fighting common health issues among men, including heart disease, diabetes, and cancer.

Let's Look at the Data

On average, the life expectancy for men, is about five years less than for women. In the United States, the average life expectancy for men is around 76 years compared to 81 years for women. Why is that?

When it comes to the leading causes of death among men, heart disease takes the top spot: it is responsible for roughly one in every four male deaths. Cancer follows closely, with lung, prostate, and colorectal cancers being the most common.

In addition, a large portion of the male population deals with a chronic disease, and in the US, about 12% of men over the age of 18 report being in "fair or poor health." Hypertension affects approximately 33% of men, and nearly 10% are living with diabetes. Obesity, a significant contributing factor to diabetes, affects around 43% of men and dramatically increases the likelihood of developing heart disease, certain cancers, and—as mentioned—diabetes. These statistics underscore the importance of regular health screenings and preventative care. By catching diseases early and making proactive lifestyle changes, men can significantly reduce the risk of developing these conditions. These sobering numbers indicate how much men stand to gain if and when they take charge of their health, if and when they start getting regular health screenings and taking preventative measures.

Mental health is another critical area that men need to address. Societal pressures and traditional notions of masculinity often prevent men from seeking help when they need it. Around 6% of the male population experiences depression, and over 3% face daily feelings of anxiety. Yet many of these men don't seek treatment due to the stigma surrounding the issue of mental health or the belief that they should "tough it out." Tragically, men are nearly four times more likely to die by suicide than women a stark reminder that mental health struggles, if left unaddressed, can have fatal consequences. Addressing these issues is crucial, and the first and foundational step is recognizing that seeking help is a sign of strength, not weakness.

Besides highlighting some of the biggest health challenges men face today, these statistics more importantly show how essential it is to break down the barriers that prevent men from taking action. As a doctor, I want you to know that taking care of your health isn't just something you should do; that kind of care is something you deserve. By focusing on regular checkups, making healthier lifestyle choices, and recognizing the importance of mental health, you can take control of your well-being and ensure a longer, more fulfilling life. Reading this book and becoming more informed is a great step. Now we'll get more specific and explore the screenings and other preventative measures you can take to mitigate your health risks and live a longer, healthier life. You owe it to yourself to make your health a priority, and the ideas in this chapter can help you do just that.

Sexual Health

Sexual health is a critical component of a person's overall well-being, yet this topic is often shrouded in silence due to societal taboos and feelings of embarrassment. For men, issues such as erectile dysfunction (ED) and sexually transmitted infections (STIs) don't only affect physical health: they also impact emotional well-being and intimate relationships. Sexual activity can also influence a man's psychological as well as physical health. Addressing all aspects of sexuality is essential for maintaining a balanced, healthy life.

Let's first consider the physical aspect of sex. During sexual activity, several key hormones are released, providing both immediate pleasure and long-term health benefits:

1. **Testosterone:** Often associated with libido, testosterone levels can increase with sexual activity. That's important because testosterone doesn't only drive a man's sexual desire; it also supports his muscle mass, bone density, and energy levels. In addition, higher levels of testosterone have been linked to an overall sense of well-being. Just remember though that too much testosterone is not a good thing and can lead to mood imbalances and blood clots.
2. **Oxytocin:** Known as the "love hormone" or "cuddle hormone," oxytocin is released during physical intimacy, especially during orgasm. It fosters bonding between partners, helps reduce stress, and strengthens emotional connections. Oxytocin is also linked to reduced fear and increased feelings of trust that nurture healthy, intimate relationships.

While sexual activity has many physical benefits, it's important to address any underlying issues that might arise, particularly when they interfere with your well-being or the dynamics of the relationship. If you're experiencing erectile dysfunction or any concerns regarding your sexual health, it's vital to seek medical advice. Not only can ED be a sign of underlying health conditions like cardiovascular disease or diabetes, but left unaddressed, it can also strain intimate relationships and affect emotional health.

It's important to understand that sexual health is more than performance or frequency; it also includes comfort, communication, and mutual satisfaction in your relationship. If you're facing challenges like ED, don't hesitate to have a conversation with your partner and your doctor. Effective treatments are available, and addressing these issues can significantly improve both your physical health and your emotional connection to your partner.

The list of benefits that sexual activity offers continues.

Cardiovascular Health:

- Men who engage in regular sexual activity have a lower risk of developing heart disease. A study published in *The American Journal of Cardiology* found that men who had sex twice or more a week had a significantly lower risk of developing cardiovascular diseases compared to men who had sex less frequently.

- Regular sexual activity is associated with reduced blood pressure. A study in the *Journal of Health and Social Behavior* concluded that sexual activity could lower systolic blood pressure.

A Boost to the Immune System:

- Engaging in sexual activity 1 to 2 times a week has been linked to higher levels of the antibody immunoglobulin A (IgA) in saliva, according to research published in *Psychological Reports*. IgA plays a critical role in immune function and can protect against common colds and other infections.

Pain Relief:

- The release of endorphins during orgasm can act as a natural pain reliever. Research indicates that sexual activity can lead to partial or complete headache relief in some migraine and cluster headache patients.

Improved Prostate Health:

- Frequent ejaculations, whether through sex, masturbation, or nocturnal emissions, may reduce the risk of prostate cancer. A landmark study in the *Journal of the American Medical Association* found that men who ejaculated 21 times or more per month had a 33% lower risk of prostate cancer then men who report fewer ejaculations.

Exercise and Weight Control:

- Sex is not a replacement for regular cardiovascular and strength training exercises, but it does burn calories. A study published in *PLOS ONE* estimated that on average, men burn 4.2 calories per minute during sexual activity, making it a form of moderate exercise.

Improved Sleep:

- The release of prolactin and oxytocin after orgasm promotes relaxation and sleepiness. Good quality sleep is linked to a host of health benefits, including improved heart health, better weight management, and reduced stress levels.

Longevity:

- Regular sexual activity might be linked to longer life. A study reported that men with a high frequency of orgasm had a 50% reduced risk of mortality over a 10-year period compared to those experiencing less frequent lower orgasms.

Erectile Dysfunction

Erectile dysfunction (ED) is a condition that affects a man's ability to achieve or maintain an erection suitable for sexual activity. This common issue impacts men worldwide, significantly affecting their confidence, relationships, and overall quality of life.

Approximately 30 million men in the United States deal with ED, and the likelihood of experiencing ED increases with age. About 40% of men are affected at age 40, and the number rises to about 70% by the age of 70. Despite its prevalence, only about a quarter of the men with ED seek treatment, often due to embarrassment or the misconception that it's a natural part of aging and nothing can be done.

To understand why ED occurs, it's helpful to know how an erection works anatomically and physiologically. In simple terms, think of the penis as a balloon that gets filled with water (in this case, blood) to become firm (erect). For the penis to fill with blood, several things need to happen:

1. **Blood Flow:** First, when a man becomes sexually aroused, his brain sends signals to the nerves in his penis. These nerves tell the blood vessels in the penis to relax, and this relaxation opens the vessels, allowing more blood to flow into the penis. To return to our analogy, turning on the hose filled the balloon with water.

2. **Blood Retention:** As the blood flows into the penis, it gets trapped in the spongelike areas called the corpora cavernosa, causing the penis to expand and become erect. The penis stays erect as long as the blood stays in the corpora cavernosa, ideally until after the sexual activity or the sexual arousal ends.

3. **Venous Closure:** As the blood is flowing into the penis, the veins that let blood out of the penis get compressed. This action helps to trap the blood inside the penis.

4. Now, if there's a problem at any stage of this process, erectile dysfunction can happen:

- **Not Enough Blood Flow:** If the blood vessels can't relax properly or if they're not healthy (maybe because of heart disease, diabetes, or smoking), not enough blood flows into the penis to make it erect.

- **Blood Doesn't Stay Trapped:** Sometimes the blood might flow into the penis, but it doesn't stay trapped there. The reason could be damaged valves that don't allow the veins to compress properly.
- **Nerve Signals Don't Work Properly:** If surgery, diabetes, or other conditions have damaged the nerves, the brain might not be able to send the right signals to the penis to start the erection process.

Causes of Erectile Dysfunction

ED can result from a combination of physical, psychological, and lifestyle factors. Physical causes can include heart disease, diabetes, high blood pressure, and obesity, all of which can affect blood flow to the penis. Psychological factors such as stress, anxiety, depression, and relationship problems can also contribute to ED. Moreover, lifestyle choices like smoking, excessive alcohol consumption, and a general lack of physical activity have been linked to the development of ED.

Natural Supplements for ED

1. **L-Arginine:** The body uses this amino acid to make nitric oxide that relaxes blood vessels and facilitates successful erections. Some studies suggest L-arginine might improve ED symptoms especially when combined with other supplements like pycnogenol.
2. **Ginseng:** Often referred to as "herbal Viagra," ginseng has been studied for its potential in improving ED. In clinical studies, red ginseng in particular has shown some promise for treating ED by enhancing penile rigidity and libido.
3. **Yohimbe:** Derived from the bark of an African evergreen tree, yohimbe has been traditionally used for sexual dysfunction. Yohimbine, the active compound, may have a positive effect on erection quality. However, it can also cause side effects like increased heart rate and blood pressure.
4. **Horny Goat Weed (Epimedium):** This herb contains icariin, a compound that acts similarly to medications used to treat ED. It's believed to help by increasing blood flow to the penis, but scientific evidence supporting its effectiveness is limited.

5. **Dehydroepiandrosterone (DHEA):** This natural hormone is produced by the adrenal glands. Supplements can be made from soy or wild yam. Some evidence suggests that DHEA supplements can help with ED especially among men with low levels of this hormone.

Hormone Health

Testosterone is often associated with male sexuality and reproduction, but it also plays a critical role in muscle mass and strength, bone density, fat distribution, red blood cell production, an overall sense of well-being, and energy levels. Testosterone levels naturally peak in a man's late teens to early twenties and start to decline, on average, by about 1% per year after the age of 30 or 40.

The decline in testosterone levels can lead to a variety of symptoms that range in severity among individuals. These symptoms can include:

- Increased abdominal fat
- Reduced muscle mass and feelings of physical weakness
- Decreased bone density, increasing the risk of osteoporosis
- Mood changes, including irritability and depression
- Fatigue and a decreased sense of well-being
- Cognitive changes, such as difficulty concentrating
- Reduced libido (sex drive) and ED

It's estimated that low testosterone affects between 2% and 6% of men, with the likelihood increasing as men age. By the age of 45, as many as 40% of men may experience testosterone levels below the optimal range for supporting well-being and overall health. It's natural for testosterone levels to decrease with age, yet those lower levels can sometimes impact energy, mood, and libido. Despite the prevalence of low testosterone, only a small percentage of men seek treatment. In fact, studies suggest that only about 5% of men with low levels of testosterone are receiving appropriate care even though treatment options are available that can significantly improve their quality of life.

Testosterone Replacement Therapy

Testosterone Replacement Therapy (TRT) addresses the symptoms of low testosterone levels in men, a condition known as hypogonadism, brings testosterone levels in the body back to a normal range. TRT can help improve symptoms such as fatigue, low libido, muscle weakness, and mood changes. The choice of treatment—including injections, patches, gels, or pellets that are placed under the skin—depends on personal preference, the severity of symptoms, and health considerations.

The Benefits of TRT

1. **Improved Energy Levels:** Many men report a significant boost in overall energy and a reduction in feelings of fatigue.
2. **Increased Muscle Mass and Strength:** TRT can help reverse the effects of muscle weakness and loss.
3. **Enhanced Mood and Greater Sense of Well-Being:** Treatment can alleviate mood swings, irritability, and depression, improving overall quality of life.
4. **Improved Libido:** Treatment can help improve sexual drive and function.
5. **Better Bone Density:** TRT can contribute to stronger bones, helping to prevent osteoporosis.

TRT: Risks and Considerations

TRT offers numerous benefits, but it's not without its risks. Potential side effects and risks include:

- Increased risk of heart-related issues, including heart attack and stroke, especially in older men or those with preexisting heart conditions
- A higher chance of developing blood clots
- Possible worsening of sleep apnea or snoring
- Skin reactions at the application site, especially with gels and patches
- The potential for stimulating the growth of existing prostate cancer, though more research is needed in this area

If you're experiencing any of these symptoms or are concerned about low testosterone, talk to your doctor about whether TRT may be a suitable option for you. A medical professional can help you weigh the benefits and the risks and then make the best decision for your health.

Health at Any Age

Understanding that your health needs change with age is crucial for maintaining long-term wellness. Each decade of a man's life brings unique health concerns that require attention and specific care strategies.

In Your 20s and 30s:

- **Alcohol and Cannabis**: When occasional alcohol or cannabis use is part of your social life, it's important to consume both in moderation. Excessive alcohol intake can lead to liver disease, heart issues, and increased blood pressure. Similarly, frequent cannabis use can impact cognitive function, memory, and mental health. Be mindful of how these substances affect your well-being and, if necessary, discuss any concerns with your healthcare provider.
- **Testicular Self-Exams**: Men should start monthly self-exams for testicular cancer in their teens and continue those exams throughout their life. To perform a self-exam, feel for any unusual lumps or changes in the size, shape, or texture of the testicles. A painless lump is often the first sign of testicular cancer, and early detection is key to effective treatment.
- **Blood Pressure Checks**: Have your blood pressure checked at least once every two years or more frequently if your doctor recommends it. The normal range is 120/80 mmHg. Check your blood pressure at home with a digital blood pressure monitor to stay on top of your health.
- **Cholesterol Screenings**: Start checking your cholesterol every 4 to 6 years. High cholesterol can increase the risk of heart disease, so managing your levels early can help prevent long-term health problems.
- **Diabetes Screening**: If your body mass index (BMI) is 25 or higher and you have other risk factors for diabetes, like family history or high blood pressure, consider getting screened for diabetes. Early detection can prevent complications down the road.
- **STI Screenings**: If you are sexually active, especially with new or multiple partners, regular STI screenings are essential for protecting your health and preventing the spread of infections. Discuss testing options with your healthcare provider.

- **Stress and Well-Being Check-Ins**: With career, relationships, and life changes in the mix, life can be stressful during your 20s and 30s. Take time to check in on your mental well-being, and if you're feeling overwhelmed or anxious, seek help from a therapist or counselor to maintain a healthy balance of work and play, and of relationships and self-care time.

In Your 40s:
- **Prostate Cancer Screening:** Talk to your doctor about whether you should have a prostate-specific antigen (PSA) test to screen for prostate cancer. Factors like family history, ethnicity, and others may influence when you start screening.
- **Eye Exams:** Get a comprehensive eye exam annually especially if you spend a lot of time in front of screens. Prolonged screen leads to eye strain. Regular checkups can detect early signs of vision issues and diseases like glaucoma or cataracts.
- **Testosterone Levels:** Consider having your testosterone level checked especially if you're experiencing fatigue, low libido, or mood changes. Testosterone naturally declines with age, and monitoring its level can help a doctor address issues related to hormone imbalances.
- **In Your 50s and After:**
- **Colorectal Cancer Screening:** Starting at age 50 or earlier if you have a family history, it's essential to get screened for colorectal cancer. Early detection is key to successful treatment, and common screening methods include colonoscopy and fecal occult blood test (FOBT). Your healthcare provider may recommend other options based on your risk factors.
- **Bone Density Test:** Men at risk for osteoporosis should consider a bone density test. Risk factors include having a family history of osteoporosis, a low-calcium or low-dairy diet, long-term steroid use, smoking, or heavy alcohol consumption. If any of these factors are present in your life, speak with your doctor about your bone health.
- **Vaccinations:** Stay up-to-date on your vaccinations, including tetanus, diphtheria, pertussis (Tdap); shingles; and pneumococcal

vaccines. Additionally, an annual flu shot is recommended for everyone especially as you age because the immune system becomes more vulnerable.

James Faces His Fears

> James, a 55-year-old mechanic in a rural town, prided himself on toughness. Frequent nighttime bathroom trips and pelvic discomfort shook him. His wife insisted on a checkup, and a PSA test flagged early prostate enlargement. James ate more tomatoes and nuts for prostate health, rode his bike daily, and opened up to his wife for support. Regular screenings kept him on track. Six months later, his symptoms eased, and he felt stronger. James even convinced his brother to get checked. Real strength meant facing fears.

Your Prostate

Prostate health is an important issue for men especially as we age. To understand prostate health, including common issues like benign prostatic hyperplasia (BPH) and prostate cancer, it helps to start with the basics of what the prostate is and how it functions.

Picture a walnut-sized gland sitting just below your bladder and surrounding the tube (urethra) that carries urine from the bladder out through the penis. This gland, part of a man's reproductive system, is the prostate. Its main job is to produce a fluid that, together with sperm from the testicles and fluids from other glands, makes up semen. This prostate fluid is important because it nourishes and, during ejaculation, transports sperm. During ejaculation, the prostate squeezes this fluid into the urethra and expels it with sperm as semen. The muscles of the prostate also help propel this seminal fluid into the urethra during ejaculation.

These muscles perform another important function: they help control the flow of urine even though the prostate is not directly part of the urinary tract. Benign Prostatic Hyperplasia (BPH) is incredibly common, affecting about 50% of men in their 50s and up to 90% of men over 80. It's not a cancerous condition, but it can affect how you urinate because that walnut-sized gland has grown bigger and started to squeeze or press on the urethra. This pressure makes it harder to urinate. Symptoms include needing to urinate often, trouble starting to urinate, or feeling like you can't fully empty your bladder.

Prostate Cancer is one of the most common cancers among men in the United States. It occurs when cells in the prostate start to grow uncontrollably. Unlike BPH, prostate cancer can spread (metastasize) to other parts of the body. Early prostate cancer is usually asymptomatic (without symptoms), which is why screening is important. According to the American Cancer Society, about 1 in 8 men will be diagnosed with prostate cancer during their lifetime, but the survival rate is promising. More than 3.1 million men in the US who have been diagnosed with prostate cancer at some point are currently alive today.

Keeping Your Prostate Healthy

Maintaining a healthy lifestyle can contribute to good prostate health. This lifestyle includes regular exercise, eating a diet rich in vegetables, maintaining a healthy weight, and not smoking. In addition, pumpkin seeds that are rich in zinc and antioxidants may support prostate health and alleviate BPH symptoms by regulating hormone levels, so you might want to sprinkle some on a salad. Lycopene, a powerful antioxidant found in tomatoes and other red fruits and vegetables, may reduce the risk of prostate cancer by lowering oxidative stress and inflammation, so include plenty of tomatoes in your diet too.

For men over a certain age or with risk factors for prostate issues, regular checkups with a healthcare provider can mean catching any problems early when they're most treatable.

You might also want to consider taking natural supplements to support prostate health:

1. **Saw Palmetto**: is often used to ease frequent urination, a symptom of benign prostatic hyperplasia (BPH). It may also inhibit enzymes that promote prostate growth.
2. **Beta-Sitosterol** can improve urinary symptoms related to BPH, such as flow rate and residual urine volume, possibly by reducing inflammation.

3. **Pygeum Africanum** is extracted from the bark of the African plum tree and used to reduce symptoms of BPH and prostatitis by minimizing inflammation and promoting toxin elimination.

Men's health deserves attention, intention, and action. Taking care of your body and mind today builds the foundation for a stronger, healthier future. Small, consistent choices add up — and they can make all the difference.

10 Ways to Enhance YOUR Health

1. Prioritize Sleep in Order to Regulate Hormones and Restore Energy

Quality sleep is one of the most powerful keys to muscle recovery, hormone regulation, and cognitive function. Yet many men sacrifice sleep for work, late-night screen time, or stress. Poor sleep can lead to lower testosterone levels, weight gain, and an increased risk of heart disease.

Here are some tips for improving sleep quality:

- Stick to a consistent bedtime.
- Keep your room cool and dark.
- Avoid screens and caffeine in the evening.
- Try magnesium or melatonin if needed.

2. Practice Mindfulness to Manage Stress and Increase Mental Clarity

Men often bottle up stress instead of finding healthy ways to manage it, leading to higher cortisol levels, anxiety, and an increased risk of heart disease. Mindfulness and meditation can help reduce stress, improve mental focus, and lower blood pressure.

These are three simple mindfulness practices:

- Take five deep breaths before reacting to stress.
- Use a meditation app for 5 to 10 minutes daily.
- Spend time in nature to reset your mind.

3. Stay Hydrated to Improve Energy Level and Performance

Proper hydration supports muscle function, digestion, and brain performance. Dehydration can lead to low energy, poor focus, and even headaches.

Here are a few hydration tips:

- Aim to drink at least 8 glasses of water per day.
- Increase your water intake if you exercise intensely or live in a hot climate.
- Add electrolytes if you sweat heavily during workouts.

4. Get Regular Checkups So You Catch Problems Early

Many men avoid doctor visits until a problem becomes serious—but don't wait! Regular checkups allow for the early detection of issues like high blood pressure, diabetes, and prostate problems.

This list of key screenings also indicates when they should start happening:

- Blood pressure & cholesterol (yearly starting at age 20)
- Diabetes screening (every 3 years starting at age 45 or, if overweight, earlier)
- Testosterone levels (if experiencing fatigue, low libido, or depression)
- Prostate health screening (starting at age 50 or, if high risk, 40)

5. Build and Maintain Strong Social Connections

Men are less likely than women to maintain close friendships, but strong social ties are key to mental health, stress reduction, and longevity. Isolation is linked to higher rates of depression and heart disease.

Find ways to stay connected:

- Join a sports league, fitness class, or community group.
- Schedule a monthly meetup with some friends.
- Prioritize quality time with your family.

6. Take Oral Hygiene Seriously (Did You Know It's Linked to Heart Health?)

Good oral hygiene is about more than fresh breath. Gum disease is linked to heart disease, inflammation, and erectile dysfunction.

Make these hygiene practices habits:

- Brush twice daily with fluoride toothpaste.
- Floss every night.
- Schedule a dental checkup twice a year.

7. Protect Your Skin to Prevent Cancer and Aging

Men are twice as likely as women to develop skin cancer due to their lower rate of sunscreen use. Regular sun exposure without protection accelerates aging, wrinkles, and skin damage.

Adopt these skin protection strategies:

- Every day—even on cloudy days—use SPF 30 or higher.
- When you're outside, wear a hat and UV-blocking sunglasses.
- Check your skin monthly for new moles or any changes.

8. Add Omega-3 Fatty Acids for Brain, Heart, and Joint Health

Omega-3s are essential fats that reduce inflammation, support brain function, and enhance heart health. They can also improve skin elasticity and boost mood.

9. Boost Zinc Intake for Testosterone and Immune Support

Zinc is crucial for testosterone production, immune function, and muscle recovery. Low levels can lead to fatigue, hair loss, and reduced strength.

10. Consider Supplements for Sexual and Prostate Health

Men's sexual health declines due to stress, poor circulation, and hormonal imbalances. Natural supplements can support circulation, endurance, and prostate function.

Here are common supplements for men's health:

- L-Arginine & Citrulline (boost nitric oxide for better circulation)
- Ginseng (enhances energy and sexual function)
- Horny Goat Weed (supports blood flow)
- Saw Palmetto (protects prostate health)

Your Action Plan: Take Control Today

1. Choose One Health Habit to Improve This Week

Building lifelong health starts with small, intentional steps. What area of your health needs the most attention right now?

- ☐ Prioritizing sleep and recovery
- ☐ Managing stress and building mental resilience
- ☐ Improving nutrition and hydration
- ☐ Increasing physical activity and strength training
- ☐ Reducing alcohol, tobacco, or other harmful habits

Write down one specific action you will take this week to improve your health:

2. Schedule Any Overdue Health Checkups

Preventative care is key to catching problems early and optimizing long-term health. When was your last checkup?

- ☐ Annual physical and blood work
- ☐ Blood pressure and cholesterol screening
- ☐ Prostate health check (starting at age 50 or, if high risk, earlier)
- ☐ Colonoscopy (starting at age 45)
- ☐ Dental exam and eye exam

3. Track Your Progress for 30 Days

Consistency leads to results. Choose one or more areas to track:

- ☐ Workouts and movement
- ☐ Sleep and recovery
- ☐ Nutrition and hydration
- ☐ Stress levels and mood
- ☐ Reduction of unhealthy habits

How will you track your progress?

- ☐ Use a fitness or health tracking app.
- ☐ Keep a simple notebook or journal.
- ☐ Look in the mirror and check in weekly with yourself. Keep yourself honest!

Two Final Thoughts: Invest in Your Health Now

- Your strength and energy, today and in the future, as well as your longevity depend on the choices you make today.
- Whatever your age or current physical condition, it's never too late to improve your health and well-being.

CHAPTER 10

THE NEXT GENERATION:

GIVING OUR CHILDREN A HEALTHY START ON A HEALTHY LIFE

Emily had an infectious laugh and a smile that could light up a room. As a high-school junior, she was active on the school's debate team and dedicated to her dream of becoming a lawyer. But lately Emily's laughter had quieted, and her smile had become less frequent. Her friends noticed her absence from social gatherings, and her grades, once a source of pride, began to slip.

At first Emily dismissed her increasing sadness and fatigue as just a phase, something all 17-year-olds go through. But as weeks turned into months, the bad days outnumbered the good. She started spending her afternoons curled up in bed, her vibrant energy replaced by a pensive gloom.

Her parents, initially attributing her changes to typical teen angst, grew concerned as Emily's condition seemed to deepen. One evening her mother found her crying in her room. Between sobs, Emily said she felt overwhelmed and hopeless, and she didn't understand why.

Recognizing the severity of her distress, Emily's parents sought help. They scheduled an appointment with a therapist who specialized in adolescent mental health. The therapist diagnosed Emily with clinical depression, a condition they explained was quite common but often misunderstood among teenagers.

Working with her therapist, Emily learned about depression, including its symptoms and underlying causes. In her twice-a-week therapy sessions, she explored her feelings in a safe environment and learned coping strategies. Her therapist also suggested integrating physical activities into her routine, improving her sleep habits, and attending a local support group for teens struggling with mental health.

Emily's road to recovery was gradual. On some days she felt she took two steps back for every step she'd taken forward, but she learned to recognize those moments as part of her healing process. When her therapist introduced her to mindfulness techniques, Emily found them particularly helpful when she found herself getting anxious. She also began documenting her thoughts and feelings in a journal, and that writing became a powerful release for her emotions.

The support from her peers also played a critical role in her recovery. As she opened up about her struggles, Emily was surprised when many of her classmates shared about their own similar experiences. This connection helped break down her feelings of isolation. The debate team also rallied around her, and their unwavering support showed her that she wasn't alone on this journey. These connections, now richer, provided Emily with a community of understanding and encouraging people who bolstered her confidence and motivated her to continue managing her depression.

If you're a parent reading this, you might recognize Emily's experience in your own child or in a teenager you know. The fact that Emily is not an outlier raises the question "What can we do to help care for the young people in our life?" That's what we'll look at in this chapter: ways to support the mental health of young people we know, foster resilience in them, and ensure they know they're never alone in their struggles.

Nurturing the Next Generation

When children are healthy, they can thrive and develop into competent, confident, and well-rounded adults. Health is essential to our children's cognitive development and emotional well-being as well as to their physical growth.

Focusing on their health when they're young helps them form habits that will serve them well throughout their lifetime, impacting everything from academic success to long-term disease prevention. Regular checkups might mean early health interventions and the opportunity to address potential issues before they become significant, setting the stage for a healthier life.

Children might not always want to eat the healthiest food, and they might prefer screen time to riding a bike, but we can always introduce them to healthier activities and practices whatever their age.

Addressing Childhood Obesity

Childhood obesity is one of the most pressing health concerns facing today's youth. According to the Centers for Disease Control and Prevention (CDC), nearly 1 in 5 children and adolescents in the US about 19.7%, or approximately 14.7 million young individuals are classified as obese. This epidemic has profound implications on their emotional well-being as well as on their physical health. Obesity in children significantly increases their risk of developing chronic conditions such as type 2 diabetes, high blood pressure, and even early-onset heart disease. Children who struggle with obesity are also more likely to experience social stigmatization that can lead to anxiety, depression, and low self-esteem.

The prevalence of obesity, however, varies by age and socioeconomic status. The rate is higher among older children and adolescents (ages 12 to 19) than younger children (ages 6 to 11) and preschoolers (ages 2 to 5). Certain demographic groups, particularly those with lower incomes and limited access to nutritious food, are disproportionately affected.

Parents can play a critical role in mitigating the risk of obesity by providing from the start a balanced diet rich in whole foods like fruits, vegetables, lean proteins, and whole grains; promoting regular physical activity (at least 60 minutes a day); and setting limits on sedentary activities like screen time. By fostering an environment that prioritizes healthy habits, parents can set their children on a path toward long-term physical and emotional health.

Nutrition

Ensuring that children receive a balanced diet rich in essential nutrients is fundamental to their growth, the strength of their immune system, and their overall health. For infants, breast milk or formula provides the necessary nutrients crucial for early development, including vital fats, proteins, and antibodies that help protect against infection. As children grow older, their dietary needs become more diverse, and it's essential to make available a wide variety of foods that contribute to their ongoing development.

A balanced diet for children should include a mix of fresh fruits and vegetables that provide essential vitamins and minerals such as Vitamin C, Vitamin A, and potassium as well as fiber. These nutrients support healthy immune function and promote eye health, skin integrity, and digestive function. Lean proteins like chicken, fish, beans, and legumes are necessary to support muscle development, tissue repair, and an effective immune system. Whole grains such as brown rice, oats, and whole wheat, for instance are excellent sources of complex carbohydrates that give children sustained energy throughout the day and provide dietary fiber that aids digestion.

Healthy fats from sources like avocados, nuts, seeds, and olive oil are essential for brain development, particularly in younger children whose brains are growing rapidly. Including dairy products like milk, yogurt, and cheese or fortified plant-based alternatives helps provide the calcium and Vitamin D crucial for strong bones and teeth.

Providing this well-balanced diet at regular mealtimes also helps children by ensuring consistent energy levels and establishing positive eating habits and routines. Structured meals complemented by healthy snacks, such as fruits, vegetables, or nuts, can help children avoid overeating as well as the consumption of nutrient-poor processed snacks that are high in sugar and saturated fats.

Consider, too, involving children in family meal preparation. Offering a variety of food options throughout the week can also make mealtime more engaging. You'll be encouraging them to develop a preference for nutritious foods and fostering a healthier relationship with eating. Educating children on the benefits of different foods and encouraging them to listen to their body's hunger and fullness cues can help build a strong foundation for lifelong healthy eating habits.

Sleep: Key to Physical and Emotional Health

At every developmental stage, getting adequate sleep is crucial to a child's health. Proper sleep supports growth, strengthens the immune system, consolidates learning, and maintains emotional balance. Infants may need up to 16 hours of sleep a day to facilitate rapid growth and brain development. Toddlers require around 11 to 14 hours, a total that can include a daytime nap.

Toddler Sleep Challenges and Solutions

As toddlers begin asserting their independence and doing so with more intense emotional responses than ever before, helping them consistently get the sleep they need can be challenging. Toddlers may have seasons of separation anxiety that make them resist going to bed, or once they are in bed, they may experience nightmares that disrupt their sleep and yours. Establishing a bedtime routine by giving toddlers a warm bath, reading a favorite bedtime story, darkening the sleep environment, making sure it's quiet and comfortable can set them up for nighttime success. The predictability of a bedtime schedule adds to a toddler's sense of security and helps prevent bedtime battles. Additionally, setting clear expectations and gently enforcing boundaries (an established bedtime, for example) can help toddlers transition more easily into sleep.

It's also important to note that toddlers are highly sensitive to the energy level of their surroundings. Having a calm and relaxed evening can help prepare them for bedtime. Avoiding stimulating activities, heavy meals, or sugar close to bedtime further supports the body's natural transition into rest.

Sleep in Adolescence: Unique Challenges and Strategies

Adolescents face unique sleep challenges. During puberty, hormonal shifts naturally alter the sleep-wake cycle, making it difficult for teens to fall asleep early and causing them to prefer later bedtimes. Since school schedules often demand early mornings, this biological shift can result in chronic sleep deprivation. Moreover, academic pressures, extracurricular activities, social obligations, and digital screen time can all interfere with an adolescent's ability to get adequate rest. The result is not only fatigue but also reduced concentration and mood swings.

To help improve your teenagers' sleep, establish or at least encourage a healthy sleep routine that balances their biological need for a later bedtime with good sleep practices. Encouraging adolescents to limit caffeine consumption, particularly in the evening, and to avoid using electronic devices at least an hour before bed can be particularly effective. Exposure to blue light from phones, tablets, and computers suppresses melatonin, the hormone responsible for regulating sleep, thus delaying the onset of sleep.

Like toddlers, adolescents also benefit from having a consistent sleep schedule even on weekends. Although teens want to sleep in, extreme variations between their schooldays and weekends can disrupt their biological clock and make it harder for them to fall asleep on weeknights. A comfortable, cool, and dark bedroom also promotes better sleep. Again like toddlers, a pre-bedtime routine that includes relaxing activities (reading, listening to calming music, or practicing mindfulness) can be a helpful signal to the body that it's time to wind down.

For both toddlers and adolescents, a consistent sleep schedule supports emotional regulation, focus, and overall well-being. Keeping that routine, managing environmental factors, and setting healthy boundaries can empower children and teenagers to develop sleep habits that contribute to their physical health, emotional stability, and academic success.

The long-term impact of ensuring that children and adolescents get the rest they need is profound, leading as it does to better mood regulation, greater resilience, better stress management, a sharper memory, improved learning, and a stronger foundation for lifelong health and well-being.

Regular Health Checkups and Developmental Screenings

Commonly referred to as well-child visits in the US, regular health checkups are essential for monitoring a child's growth and developmental progress. These visits give healthcare providers an opportunity to detect potential health issues early on, administer vaccinations, and advise parents about upcoming developmental stages. Here's what typically occurs during these visits:

- **Physical Examinations:** The doctor will measure height, weight, and body mass index (BMI) to assess physical growth patterns and examine the heart, lungs, abdomen, skin, and neurological functions

to detect any abnormalities. The doctor will also perform a visual and physical examination to assess the child's overall health.
- **Developmental Screenings:** This assessment of cognitive, behavioral, and learning aspects will help ensure that children are meeting developmental milestones appropriate for their age.
- **Sensory Screenings:** Regular vision and hearing tests are crucial for detecting sensory impairments that could affect a child's ability to learn and interact with their environment.
- **Vaccinations:** Per the schedule, the healthcare provider will advise about and/or administer vaccinations to protect against various diseases.
- **Parental Guidance:** Parents may receive information about nutrition, sleep, safety, and what developmental markers to expect in the coming months

Vaccinations

Vaccinations are a safe and effective way to protect against serious diseases throughout life. Staying on schedule with recommended vaccines from infancy through adolescence helps build strong immunity and prevent illness.

Some vaccines, like those for measles, mumps, rubella (MMR), polio, and DTaP (diphtheria, tetanus, and pertussis), are commonly required for school entry in most states. Others, such as the HPV and meningococcal vaccines, are strongly recommended during adolescence to protect against future health risks.

Not all vaccinations are mandatory, and recommendations may vary based on age, health status, and location. Always consult your doctor to understand what's best for you or your child.

Common Childhood Illnesses and Conditions

Since their immune systems are still developing and because they're with groups of people in schools and on playgrounds, children are especially prone to certain illnesses and conditions. This section provides an overview of some of the most common childhood ailments including colds, flu, allergies, asthma, and skin conditions along with guidance about home care and when to consult healthcare professionals.

Colds: According to the CDC, most children experience 6 to 8 colds each year. Symptoms typically include a runny nose, cough, mild fever, and fatigue. Usually caused by viruses, colds spread easily in places where children congregate, such as schools and daycare centers. Although colds are generally mild, they can make children uncomfortable and affect their daily activities.

More severe than the common cold, the **flu** (influenza) is characterized by fever, chills, body aches, fatigue, and respiratory symptoms. Especially in young children, this contagious respiratory illness can lead to serious complications, such as pneumonia and bronchitis. Annual flu vaccines are recommended for children 6 months and older to prevent this potentially serious illness.

If they're not properly managed, **food allergies** can pose serious health risks. Symptoms can range from mild (such as rashes and itching) to severe (like anaphylaxis). It's essential for parents to identify and minimize exposure to known allergens to prevent allergic reactions.

A chronic condition that affects the airways in the lungs, **asthma** can lead to difficulty breathing, wheezing, coughing, and tightness in the chest. According to the American Lung Association, approximately 1 in 12 children in the US has asthma. This condition can be triggered by allergens, respiratory infections, cold air, and physical activity. Managing asthma involves avoiding triggers and using prescribed medications, such as inhalers, to keep the airways open and reduce inflammation.

Tips for Home Care

- For Colds and Flu: Help the child stay hydrated. Drinking plenty of fluids helps to thin mucus and keep the throat moist. Using saline nasal drops can relieve nasal congestion and make breathing easier, and that's especially important during naps and at night. Keeping the child comfortable and encouraging rest is crucial for recovery. Using a humidifier to add moisture to the air can help ease congestion and coughing, and offering warm soups and broths can provide comfort as well as hydration.

- For Asthma: Follow the asthma action plan prescribed by the child's healthcare provider, a plan that probably includes using inhalers and other medications to control symptoms and prevent attacks. Remove known triggers, such as pet dander, mold, and dust mites, from the home environment to help reduce asthma symptoms. Encourage regular use of preventative inhalers and ensure quick access to rescue inhalers during an asthma attack.

When to Seek Professional Medical Advice

- **For Colds and Flu**: Seek medical attention if the child has difficulty breathing, symptoms last more than 10 days, or a fever runs higher than 100.4°F in infants under 3 months. These symptoms can indicate a more serious condition that requires professional evaluation and treatment. Persistent symptoms, such as a prolonged cough or high fever, can lead to complications, so timely medical intervention is crucial.

- **For Asthma**: Immediate medical help is necessary if the child exhibits signs of an asthma attack that doesn't improve with the prescribed medication. Symptoms such as severe shortness of breath, wheezing, and a rapid increase in the use of rescue inhalers indicate that the asthma is not under control, and urgent medical attention may be required. Asthma attacks can be life-threatening if they aren't treated promptly, so recognizing these signs and seeking emergency care is vital.

Physical Activity and Play

Physical activity is a crucial element of a healthy childhood, contributing significantly to the physical, emotional, and cognitive development of children. Physical activity helps to build strong bones, muscles, and joints, and it supports cardiovascular fitness, helps regulate weight, and can decrease the risk of developing chronic health conditions such as type 2 diabetes, obesity, and heart disease later in life.

- According to the Centers for Disease Control and Prevention (CDC), children and adolescents aged 6 to 17 years should engage in at least 60 minutes of moderate to vigorous physical activity daily.

- Most of that 60 minutes or more per day should be either moderate or vigorous aerobic activity. Examples include cycling, swimming, dance, and organized sports like soccer or basketball.
- Include muscle-strengthening activities in the daily 60 minutes at least 3 days a week. Activities that build muscle include gymnastics, climbing trees, or playing on playground equipment.
- Bone-strengthening activities should also be included at least 3 days a week, and the child's aerobic and muscle-strengthening activities may already be strengthening bones. Examples include jumping rope, running, and sports that involve jumping or rapid changes in direction.

The Benefits for Emotional and Social Development

In addition to being crucial for physical health, active play contributes to the emotional and social development of children. It provides a natural setting for children to express themselves, follow their imaginations, and navigate emotions and relationships. During play, children learn essential social skills. They cooperate, follow rules, negotiate for fairness, and learn to share. Playing with others helps children develop communication skills, understand the value of teamwork, and make friends, and all three of those contribute to healthy self-esteem. Incorporating physical activity and play into daily routines is essential for holistic child development.

So, as parents, we need to provide our children with opportunities for active play. Play dates count, but also encourage your child to join clubs and get involved in activities they enjoy. Gymnastics, dance, swimming, and drama can involve games and physical expression that get children moving. Don't push your children into sports simply because that's an obvious opportunity for physical activity. Finding something that captures their interest is key to nurturing their physical and emotional development.

Mental Health

Many parents tell me that they worry about their children's mental health, and it's great that we are now able to have that conversation more freely. The discussion is important because as with physical health issues, early intervention in mental health concerns can prevent more severe issues later in life. So what can parents watch out for and do to protect their children's mental health?

Children often exhibit signs of mental health issues differently from adults, and these signs can vary by age:

- **Anxiety** in children may present as excessive worry about routine activities, and their worry can often be accompanied by physical symptoms like headaches or stomachaches. According to the CDC, approximately 4.4 million children aged 3 to 17 years have been diagnosed with anxiety.

- **Depression** might not always appear as sadness; instead, it can manifest as irritability, changes in eating or sleeping patterns, or a loss of interest in activities the child once enjoyed. Again from the CDC, about 1.9 million children aged 3 to 17 years have been diagnosed with depression.

- **Behavioral disorders** may involve ongoing patterns of uncontrolled anger, defiance, or vindictiveness toward authority figures.

To support children struggling with mental health issues or to prevent it in the first place parents can do the following:

- **Create a supportive environment**: Open communication is crucial. Children should feel safe to express their thoughts and feelings without fear of judgment or punishment.

- **Establish routines**: The sense of security and predictability that routines provide is especially comforting for children who are dealing with anxiety.

- **Use positive reinforcement**: To encourage good behavior and build self-esteem, focus on effort and personal improvement rather than on just the outcomes of a child's behavior and effort.

- **Teach coping skills**: Techniques such as deep breathing, mindfulness, and talking about their feelings can help children manage stress.

- **Shield children from excessive stress**: Minimize their exposure to family conflicts, adult concerns, and inappropriate media content.

- **Seek professional support**: If your child's symptoms persist or are severe, consulting with a psychologist or psychiatrist specializing in pediatric mental health is advisable. Collaborating with education professionals can help ensure that children receive the support they need at school.

- **Encourage social interaction**: Activities involving peer interaction help improve social skills and emotional resilience. Children with an active social life tend to exhibit greater mental health than their less social peers. Encourage your child or teen to find an activity they're interested in whether it's sports, music, or drama and then help them get involved in it. This social interaction will foster personal growth and interpersonal connections.

By recognizing early signs of mental health issues and taking proactive steps, parents can significantly influence their children's mental well-being and help them grow into well-adjusted adults.

Sophie's New Balance

> Sophie, a 14-year-old teen, was glued to her phone clocking about 6 hours daily on social media. She got moody, gained weight, and had headaches. Her pediatrician linked it to screen time and mild depression. Sophie joined a school dance club, helped cook veggie-packed dinners, and used an app to cut social media to 1 hour. She met weekly with a school counselor. Two months later, her headaches faded, she smiled more, and dancing became her escape. Her family started dancing together, making home warmer.

Screen Time and Social Media

In the digital age, children are increasingly exposed to screens and social media. These platforms can offer solid educational content as well as opportunities for social connection, but limits are essential. Excessive screen time and unregulated social media use have raised concerns regarding their impact on children's mental, emotional, and physical health.

"Screen time" refers to the amount of time spent using devices with screens, such as smartphones, tablets, computers, and televisions. The American

Academy of Pediatrics (AAP) recommends that children under 18 months avoid screen time other than video-chatting. Children aged 2 to 5 years should limit screen use to 1 hour per day of high-quality programs. For children 6 years and older, parents need to enforce consistent limits on the time spent using media and the types of media being viewed.

Effects of Screen Time

Screen time on television, tablets, and smartphones adds up surprisingly quickly in the course of a day, and the medical community is beginning to see the physical and emotional impact that this extended screen time has on children and teenagers. Its hard but the goal should be to limit children's recreational screen use to no more than 1 hour per day.

Parents as well as their older children and their teenagers need to be aware of some specific effects of extended screen use:

- **Vision Problems:** Extended screen time can lead to digital eye strain, characterized by dry eyes, headaches, and blurred vision. A study in the journal *Pediatrics* found that children who spend more than 2 hours a day on screens are at a higher risk of experiencing eye discomfort.

- **Obesity:** Screen time is often a sedentary activity associated with snacking and poor dietary choices. The CDC reports that children who watch more than 2 hours of television per day have a higher propensity for being overweight.

- **Sleep Disruption:** The blue light emitted by screens can interfere with the production of melatonin, the hormone that regulates sleep-wake cycles. Research indicates that children who use devices before bedtime are more likely to suffer from sleep disturbances.

- **Attention Issues:** High amounts of screen time have been linked to a child's shorter attention span and a greater struggle to concentrate. Children who spend more than 2 hours per day on screens also score lower on aptitude tests.

- **Increased Anxiety and Depression:** Excessive use of social media can increase feelings of inadequacy, anxiety, and depression. Studies have shown that excess use of social media decreases one's sense of self-worth.

- **Social Skills Development:** Overreliance on digital communication can hinder the development of the face-to-face social skills critical to children's growth into adults who are productive members of society.

The Impact of Social Media

As we looked at in previous chapters, social media can impact the health and the sense of well-being of all of us. That impact is more profound on children and teenagers, too often negatively affecting their understanding of relationships and their sense of self-worth. Some online groups provide a space for expression and community-building, but the flip side is, these groups can also expose children to cyberbullying and unrealistic life comparisons:

Cyberbullying: The anonymity of the internet can lead to harsh interactions that would probably not occur in person. Research shows that 37% of young people between the ages of 12 and 17 have been bullied online.

Body Image Issues: Particularly among teenagers, the constant exposure to edited and curated images can create unrealistic standards of physical beauty. Studies show a correlation between social media use and body dissatisfaction, eating disorders, and low self-esteem.

FOMO (Fear of Missing Out): Social media can exacerbate feelings of anxiety when children compare their lives to the idealized experiences posted by others. Social media also exacerbates the feelings that come when they see the parties, activities, and fun that they were excluded from. Research finds a direct association between the time spent on social media and increased FOMO and negative feelings about oneself.

What Can Parents Do to Help?

Screens and social media are integral parts of modern life, and as parents we need to balance our children's screen time with healthy activities. Open dialogue is crucial for achieving this balance for our children:

- **Set Clear Boundaries:** Establish and enforce rules for how much screen time you will allow. Also ensure that screens are turned off at least one hour before bedtime so children can wind down.

- **Encourage Physical Activity:** Make sure your children have plenty of opportunities for the physical play and outside activities essential for their physical health and social development. Children should be outdoors as much as possible.
- **Monitor Content:** Be aware of what your children are watching and using on their devices. Use parental controls if necessary and always discuss the content with them.
- **Educate Children about Online Interactions:** Teach your children about the potential ramifications of online interactions, the permanence of the digital footprint, and the importance of showing kindness and empathy online.
- **Promote Open Communication:** Encourage your children to talk with you about their online experiences and resulting feelings. Having an open line of communication can help parents detect early signs of cyberbullying or other online issues.

Talking to Adolescents about Their Health

In this critical period of life marked by rapid physical, emotional, and social changes, many adolescents find it challenging to maintain both physical activity and overall health. Nearly 50% of girls drop out of sports during adolescence, yet rising obesity rates among teenagers highlight the importance of encouraging healthy habits during this stage of life. Addressing these concerns from declining participation in sports to rising rates of inactivity, weight gain, and mental health struggles can help parents better support their children.

During this period, adolescents often deal with heightened emotions and mood swings due to hormonal changes. They also form stronger, more complex friendships and may start experiencing romantic feelings. Their increasing desire for independence can sometimes lead to conflicts with parents. Staying involved in physical activities whether through organized sports, dance, martial arts, outdoor adventures, or simply regular movement like biking or walking with friends can help adolescents manage stress, boost their mood, and provide a healthy outlet for their energy and emotions.

Ideally, parents began educating children about puberty before the physical changes started. That education helps adolescents to understand beforehand what changes to expect and to be reassured that what they're experiencing is normal. Also discussing menstrual health with girls and basic hygiene with both boys and girls are also essential aspects of self-care during puberty.

Adolescents often face pressure from peers and media to look or to act a certain way, resulting in body image issues when they feel they don't measure up. Encouraging positive self-talk, focusing on body functionality over appearance, and celebrating diverse body types can help promote a teenager's healthy body image.

At a certain point adolescents will start making decisions about their lifestyle, including diet, physical activity, and sleep. Parents need to provide the food required to support their teens' growth, get the teens involved in menu planning, shopping, and food preparation, and ensure meals contain enough protein and vegetables for their growing bodies. (And, parents, your teens might need more food than you yourselves do, so be ready for that.) Encouraging healthy choices about diet as well as exercise and sleep is crucial. So is vigilance for signs of eating disorders on the part of educators and parents. These disorders commonly emerge during adolescence, and professional help is sometimes needed.

Discussions about the risks associated with tobacco, alcohol, and drug use are essential because these substances can be particularly harmful to the developing adolescent brain. By providing accurate information and supportive guidance, parents can help adolescents make informed decisions that protect their health and well-being.

Addressing Adolescent Mental Health

As adolescents navigate the complexities of their developmental stage, they face unique challenges that can impact their mental health. In fact, mental health disorders often first emerge during adolescence. According to the World Health Organization, one in six people aged 10 to 19 years experiences a mental health condition, with anxiety and depression being among the most common. In the United States, the National Institute of Mental Health reports that major depressive episodes affect approximately 13.3% of adolescents aged 12 to 17, while the American Psychological Association (APA) notes that about 20% of teenagers experience depression before reaching adulthood. Additionally, anxiety disorders affect 31.9% of teenagers, highlighting the critical need for focused mental health interventions during this stage of life.

What can we do to best support our teens at this time, and what do we need to look out for? Again, open communication is essential: our teens should feel safe expressing their feelings and seeking help from us when they need it. We parents can educate ourselves about mental health so that we are able to recognize signs that our teens are struggling. This education can also help us to create an environment where conversations about mental health are normalized. This proactive approach can help destigmatize mental health issues and make adolescents feel comfortable accessing resources.

- Symptoms of adolescent **depression** may include persistent sadness, irritability, a withdrawal from previously enjoyed activities, changes in eating and sleeping patterns, and sometimes thoughts of self-harm or suicide. Parents should look out for these signs and respond with empathy, offer support, and seek professional help if needed.
- **Anxiety** can manifest as generalized anxiety disorder, social anxiety disorder, panic attacks, and phobias. Common symptoms include excessive worry, nervousness, and physical signs like heart palpitations and sweating. Creating a supportive space where teens can openly discuss their worries and concerns is vital.
- **Eating disorders** like anorexia nervosa, bulimia nervosa, and binge eating disorder can develop or intensify during adolescence. These disorders are characterized by an unhealthy focus on weight, body shape, and food that severely impacts health. Parents can support their teens by examining their own messaging and attitudes around food and body image. Encouraging a balanced approach to eating, focusing on health rather than appearance, and avoiding negative comments about body weight either their own or their child's can create a more positive environment that helps prevent these issues or allows them to be more readily addressed.

By being observant, creating an open line of communication, and seeking professional help when necessary, parents can provide the support that their adolescents need to navigate this challenging period of life and protect their mental health.

How Can We Help?

As parents, we may often worry about our teens' mental health, so what can we do to support them? Whether helping them prepare for challenges before they arise or offering support when they're struggling, we can make a significant difference in their well-being. Other family members, friends, and educational institutions may also offer assistance and support. Creating environments and offering opportunities for relationships where adolescents feel safe, supported, and understood can greatly impact their mental health for the better.

- **Encourage Healthy Habits**: Regular physical activity, adequate sleep, and balanced nutrition are essential for improving mental health. (Physical activity in particular effectively reduces symptoms of depression and anxiety.) Make it a priority to incorporate these healthy habits into your family's routine.
- **Teach Coping Mechanisms**: Helping adolescents learn ways to handle stress ways like mindfulness, meditation, and cognitive-behavioral techniques can empower them to manage their mental health. Modeling these behaviors yourself can reinforce their importance.
- **Access Professional Help**: When necessary, help your teen access mental health professionals such as counselors, psychologists, or psychiatrists. School-based mental health services can also play a crucial role in a teen's life. Parents can advocate for these resources if they aren't already available.
- **Reduce Stigma Through Education**: Providing our teens with information about mental health can demystify these conditions and help remove any stigma surrounding them. Parents can start conversations at home, and schools and communities can offer the support of resources and programs that promote mental health awareness. Encouraging open discussions makes it easier for adolescents to seek help when they need it.

Raising a healthy next generation doesn't start when kids are teenagers it starts when they're toddlers watching what we do, listening to what we say, and learning what we value. The habits, mindsets, and priorities we model early on shape how they will care for themselves long after they leave our homes. Every healthy meal, every walk outside, every honest conversation about emotions are investments in their future. Our greatest legacy is raising kids who understand health, live it with confidence, and carry those lessons forward to the next generation.

10 Ways to Support the Next Generation

1. Foster Open and Honest Communication

Young people need a judgment-free space where they feel safe to express thoughts, emotions, and concerns. If they fear criticism or dismissal, they'll stop sharing with us and look elsewhere sometimes to unreliable sources for answers.

Create a safe space:

- Be approachable: Show curiosity instead of lecturing.
- Ask open-ended questions, not ones that can be answered yes or no.
- Be creative: "How was your day?" can feel cliched and empty. Instead, ask, "What was something that surprised you today?"
- Validate your teen's emotions: Avoid saying and even implying, "That's not a big deal." Instead say, "That sounds frustrating. Want to talk about it?"

2. Teach Balanced Nutrition and Healthy Habits

Children and young adults develop lifelong eating habits based on what they see at home. Poor nutrition contributes to mood swings, poor focus, and long-term health risks like obesity and diabetes.

Guide children and young adults toward better choices:

- Lead by example: Eat the way you want your children to eat.
- Teach the why: Explain how food affects energy, focus, and emotional balance.
- Make small swaps: Replace sugary drinks with flavored water or fresh fruit.
- Encourage independence: Let your children help choose and cook healthy meals.

3. Support Their Physical and Mental Well-Being

Physical activity is key for both physical and mental health. It improves focus, mood, and self-esteem while reducing anxiety and depression.

Encourage movement without making it a chore:

- Make movement social: Sports, group activities, and family outings work best.
- Give children options: Not every kid likes traditional sports. Encourage dance, martial arts, hiking, or skateboarding.
- Set limits on screen time: Balance tech time with active play or outdoor activities.
- Mental health also matters:
- Teach mindfulness or deep breathing for stress.
- Encourage journaling for self-reflection.
- Normalize therapy and counseling as a positive tool, not a last resort.

4. Set Boundaries on Technology and Social Media

Today's children and teens are the first fully digital generation. Technology is essential, but excessive screen time leads to sleep problems, anxiety, and unrealistic comparisons.

Create a healthy tech balance:

- Set screen-free zones: Make it a family policy to not have phones at the dinner table or use them before bed.
- Encourage creative use of tech over passive use: Get kids involved in video editing, coding, or content creation instead of endless scrolling.
- Monitor children's use social media use. Discuss cyberbullying and online safety with them.

5. Teach Stress Management and Resilience

Life is stressful, and coping skills are not intuitive: they must be taught. Help young people develop tools to navigate life's challenges and setbacks.

Build resilience:

- Model problem-solving: Talk about your own challenges and how you worked through them.
- Teach delayed gratification: The rewards of hard work aren't always immediate, but they're always worth the wait.

- Encourage a growth mindset: Reframe failure as an opportunity to learn.
- Provide healthy coping mechanisms: Exercise, deep breathing, art, and music are some good options.
- Help children identify the stress-management technique they will use the next time they feel overwhelmed.

6. Guide Children in Building Healthy Relationships

Relationships whether with friends, family, or romantic partners are crucial to emotional development. To set them up for positive relational experiences, guide young people in setting boundaries, understanding consent, and recognizing toxic behavior.

Consider these approaches:

- Discuss red flags in friendships and dating: Control, disrespect, and manipulation are three examples.
- Model healthy conflict resolution: Children learn from how you handle disagreements.
- Emphasize mutual respect: Both parties in a relationship deserve to be heard and valued.

7. Provide Regular Medical and Preventative Care

Many young people avoid doctor visits until they are sick. Teach them that routine checkups are part of ensuring lifelong health.

Prioritize regular care:

- Annual physicals: Stay on top of blood pressure, any changes in vision, and growth markers.
- Vaccinations: Keep up with recommended schedules.
- Mental health check-ins: Depression and anxiety often start in adolescence.
- Reproductive health: Discuss puberty, sexual health, and contraception in an honest, nonjudgmental way.

8. Encourage Financial and Life Skills Early On

Many young adults leave home without basic life skills, among them budgeting, cooking, self-care, and taking personal responsibility. These skills are just as essential as academics if not more so.

Teach your children what they need to know and do in everyday life. Prepare them for adulting!

- Budgeting and saving: Explain credit, debt, saving, and financial planning.
- Basic cooking skills: Healthy eating starts at home.
- Time management: Balancing school, work, and social life is a skill developed over time and with practice.
- Self-advocacy: Teach your children and model how to schedule their own appointments, make informed decisions, and take charge of real-life responsibilities.

9. Keep the Conversation about Mental Health Going

The stigma around mental health is fading, but many young people still feel ashamed or afraid to ask for help.

Provide support:

- Normalize talking about feelings and emotions.
- Emphasize that seeking help is a strength, not a weakness.
- Offer mental health resources like books, podcasts, or professional contacts.

10. Teach Risk Awareness and Safety

Young people take more risks than adults because their brains are still developing decision-making skills. Help them make informed choices instead of fear-based ones.

Be sure to discuss these key topics:

- Safe driving habits: Avoid distractions, speeding, and impaired driving.
- Substance use: Talk honestly about consequences rather than just saying, "Don't do it."

- Sexual health and consent: Have honest, clear conversations about respect and protection.

You may have noticed there's no pre-filled action plan in this section—and that's intentional. Every child is different, and the best way to support the next generation depends on their age, needs, and your family dynamic. Instead, take a moment to create your own three-point action plan using the 10 Ways to Support the Next Generation as a guide. Tailor it to your child's stage of life, and commit to steps that feel meaningful, realistic, and lasting.

CHAPTER 11

AFTER YOU CLOSE THE BOOK:

LIVING YOUR HEALTHIEST LIFE

As we close this book, let's reflect on the journey we've taken together. Throughout *YOU Are the New Prescription*, we've explored what it means to lead a healthier, more fulfilling life. From understanding the basics of mental and physical health to diving deep into the nuances of preventative care and emotional well-being, we've covered a vast range of information.

We first laid a strong foundation with the fundamentals of physical health. You read about the critical importance of cardiovascular health and steps to take to keep your heart strong. Understanding the importance of dietary choices, regular physical activity, and stress management techniques serves as your first line of defense against the leading causes of illness and death around the world.

Next we gave mental health the attention it deserves and reflected on its role in overall health. We delved into strategies for maintaining mental agility and emotional resilience. Knowing how to manage stress, combat anxiety, and foster a positive mental outlook means being equipped with a healthy mind as we face life's challenges.

Embracing the present moment was highlighted as a transformative practice for personal well-being. Cultivating a state of awareness can enhance your connection to the here and now, leading to a richer, more fulfilling life. This practice not only improves mental clarity but also contributes to emotional and physical health by reducing stress and its many associated risks.

Perhaps one of the most empowering aspects of our journey was addressing our unhealthy habits. Smoking, excessive alcohol consumption, unhealthy eating, and sedentary lifestyles are some of the topics we tackled. As we explored practical methods for breaking free from these chains, we emphasized the value of making gradual changes rather than drastic and abrupt adjustments. We also reminded you to extend yourself compassion rather than sit in guilt as you work on replacing unhealthy habits with healthy ones.

Advocating a holistic approach to health, we looked at the way a human being's physical, mental, and emotional parts are inextricably linked to each other. You learned, for instance, that treating the body well supports mental clarity and that nurturing the mind can enhance physical vitality. Recognizing this interconnectedness of the physical, mental, and emotional parts of ourselves is key to healthy living. Our physical health influences our mental state, our mental resilience affects our emotional stability, and all these aspects impact our ability to live fully and actively in the present moment. When you understand these connections, you can see why adjustments in one area can bring about positive changes in other aspects of your life.

Continue to educate yourself. Attend health seminars, subscribe to wellness newsletters, and participate in community health initiatives. Dive deeper into subjects like nutrition, exercise, and mental health through trusted resources from government-backed organizations like the Centers for Disease Control and Prevention (CDC), the National Institutes of Health (NIH), and the U.S. Department of Agriculture (USDA). And if you're looking for even more, I've included a list of recommended books, websites, and tools in the Resources section at the back of this book. The more you learn, the more confident and empowered you'll feel to make choices that support your health — and inspire those around you to do the same.

As we conclude our journey through this book, I want to extend my heartfelt thanks to you for joining us. I hope you've been both encouraged and prepared to continue on this path toward better health and wellness. It's been a privilege to share this information with you, and I hope it has inspired you to take meaningful action in your life.

After all, the end of this book is the beginning of a new chapter of your journey. Keep learning, stay curious, and engage with a community that supports your continued growth. Celebrate your successes, learn from the challenges, and remember that every small step you take is part of your larger journey toward health and happiness. Celebrate your successes, learn from the challenges, and remember that every small step you take is part of your larger journey toward health and happiness.

At the end of the day, the most powerful prescription isn't something you pick up from a pharmacy. It's the daily choices you make to move, to nourish, to rest, to grow. This is your life. This is your health.

YOU are the new prescription.

PART IV
TOOLS TO TAKE WITH YOU

APPENDIX A

The Ramaswamy Supplement Stack List

- **Omega-3 fatty acids** support brain function and heart health as well as reduce inflammation.
- **Vitamin D** is essential for bone health, immune function, and mood regulation.
- **Magnesium** helps with muscle relaxation, sleep quality, and cardiovascular health.
- **Coenzyme Q10 (CoQ10)** supports heart health, energy production, and cellular function.
- **Probiotics** promote gut health, digestion, and the immune system.
- **B-Complex Vitamins** improve energy levels, brain function, and the production of red blood cells.
- **Zinc** boosts immune function, aids the healing of wounds, and supports skin health.
- **Collagen** enhances skin elasticity, strengthens joints, and supports hair and nail growth.
- **Turmeric (Curcumin)** serves as a powerful anti-inflammatory and antioxidant for joint and brain health.
- **L-Arginine** improves circulation, supports cardiovascular health, and boosts nitric oxide levels.

APPENDIX B

Key Health Markers to Track for Optimal Wellness

TIER 1: ESSENTIAL TESTS FOR GENERAL HEALTH

(Recommended for routine health maintenance and disease prevention)

1. Metabolic Health & Blood Sugar

- **Fasting Blood Glucose** screens for diabetes and insulin resistance. (Normal: <100 mg/dL)
- **Hemoglobin A1C (HbA1c)** measures average blood sugar over 3 months. (Normal: <5.7%)
- **Insulin Levels** assesses insulin resistance and metabolic health. (Optimal: <10 µU/mL)
- **Cardiovascular & Heart Health**
- **Lipid Panel (Total Cholesterol, LDL, HDL, Triglycerides)** assesses risk of heart disease.
- **High-Sensitivity C-Reactive Protein (hs-CRP)** detects systemic inflammation linked to heart disease. (Optimal: <1 mg/L)
- **Kidney & Liver Function**
- **Creatinine & Estimated Glomerular Filtration Rate (eGFR)** measures kidney function.
- **Liver Enzymes (AST, ALT, ALP, GGT)** indicate liver stress and disease.

4. Hormonal & Nutrient Health

- **Thyroid Panel (TSH, Free T3, Free T4)** assesses thyroid function and metabolism.
- **Vitamin D (25-hydroxyVitamin D)** is essential for immunity, bone health, and overall function. (Optimal: 40-60 ng/mL)
- **Vitamin B12 & Folate** are key to nerve function, healthy red blood cells, and DNA synthesis.

TIER 2: ADVANCED BIOMARKERS FOR LONGEVITY & PERFORMANCE

(For those optimizing longevity, athletic performance, and long-term disease prevention)

5. Metabolic & Energy Optimization

- **HOMA-IR** evaluates insulin resistance and metabolic flexibility.
- **Adiponectin & Leptin Levels** assess fat metabolism and energy regulation.

6. Cardiovascular Longevity & Inflammation

- **Apolipoprotein B (ApoB)** is a stronger predictor of cardiovascular risk than LDL alone.
- **Lipoprotein(a) (Lp(a))** offers a genetic risk marker for cardiovascular disease.
- **Pulse Wave Velocity (PWV)** measures arterial stiffness, a key predictor of cardiovascular aging.
- **Muscle, Strength, & Physical Longevity**
- **VO2 Max & Resting Heart Rate** measures cardiovascular fitness and longevity.
- **Grip Strength Test** is a well-researched predictor of longevity and functional aging.
- **D3-Creatine Dilution Test** serves as a precise test for total muscle mass, relevant for aging and strength.

8. Brain & Cognitive Function

- **Omega-3 Index** measures these fatty acids that have been linked to reduced cognitive decline, brain health, and neuroprotection.
- **Brain-Derived Neurotrophic Factor (BDNF)** assesses the presence of this gene that supports neuroplasticity, memory, and brain longevity.

TIER 3: SPECIALIZED & ENVIRONMENTAL TESTING

(For those interested in deeper insights, disease risk, and environmental exposures)

9. **Cellular Aging & Epigenetics**

- **DNA Methylation & Epigenetic Age Testing** determines the gap between biological age and chronological age.
- **Telomere Length Testing** measures cellular aging and longevity potential.

10. **Oxidative Stress & Inflammation**

- **8-Hydroxy-2'-deoxyguanosine (8-OHdG)** provides a biomarker for oxidative DNA damage.
- **F2-Isoprostanes** can assess oxidative stress and lipid peroxidation.

11. **Gut Health & Digestive Function**

- **Comprehensive Stool Analysis** evaluates gut microbiome, digestion, and inflammation.
- **Zonulin & Intestinal Permeability Markers** detect "leaky gut" syndrome.

12. **Heavy Metals & Environmental Toxins**

- **Heavy Metal Panel (Lead, Mercury, Arsenic, Cadmium, Aluminum)** identifies toxic metal exposure.
- **Glyphosate & Environmental Toxin Testing** measures exposure to pesticides and chemicals.

APPENDIX C

The Ramaswamy Daily Health Routine

A simple breakdown of daily habits for optimal health and longevity

Morning Routine

- Hydration: Electrolytes, Lemon Water
- Morning Sun Exposure: Circadian Rhythm Regulation
- Movement: Stretching, Mobility, Walking
- Mindfulness: Breathing, Meditation, Gratitude

Daily Essentials

- Optimal Timing of Meals & Fasting Considerations
- Prioritizing Whole Nutrient-Dense Foods
- Smart Timing of Supplements

Evening Routine

- Winding Down for Sleep: No Screens, Blue Light Management
- Nighttime Supplements & Relaxation Practices

APPENDIX D

Resources to Keep YOU Moving Forward

Learning doesn't stop when you finish this book — in fact, that's where real change begins. I've put together a curated list of trusted resources to help you dive deeper, stay curious, and keep building a life of health and vitality. These books and websites offer practical guidance and evidence-based information you can return to again and again.

Further Recommended Reading

Books that complement the ideas in this book and offer powerful insights into health, behavior, longevity, and well-being:

- How Not to Die by Dr. Michael Greger
- Atomic Habits by James Clear
- Spark: The Revolutionary New Science of Exercise and the Brain by Dr. John Ratey
- The Blue Zones by Dan Buettner
- Why We Sleep by Dr. Matthew Walker
- Outlive: The Science and Art of Longevity by Dr. Peter Attia
- Younger Next Year by Chris Crowley and Dr. Henry S. Lodge
- The Body Keeps the Score by Dr. Bessel van der Kolk
- Lifespan: Why We Age—and Why We Don't Have To by Dr. David Sinclair
- Grit: The Power of Passion and Perseverance by Angela Duckworth
- The End of Alzheimer's by Dr. Dale Bredesen

Trusted Websites

Government-backed organizations with clear, science-based information:

- Centers for Disease Control and Prevention (CDC) — www.cdc.gov
- National Institutes of Health (NIH) — www.nih.gov
- U.S. Department of Agriculture (USDA) — www.nutrition.gov
- National Institute on Aging (NIA) — www.nia.nih.gov
- Office of Disease Prevention and Health Promotion — www.health.gov
- Environmental Working Group (EWG) — www.ewg.org

BIBLIOGRAPHY

Understanding Mental Health: Nurturing your Inner Strength

American Psychiatric Association. (2020). Diagnostic and statistical manual of mental disorders (5th ed.). Arlington, VA: American Psychiatric Publishing.

Centers for Disease Control and Prevention (CDC). (2021). Mental health statistics in the U.S. Retrieved from https://www.cdc.gov

Harvard Medical School. (2021). The impact of stress on mental health. Boston: Harvard Health Publishing.

Mayo Clinic. (2021). Anxiety disorders: Symptoms and treatments. Retrieved from https://www.mayoclinic.org

National Alliance on Mental Illness (NAMI). (2021). Mental health by the numbers. Retrieved from https://www.nami.org

National Institute of Mental Health (NIMH). (2021). Prevalence of mental health disorders. Retrieved from https://www.nimh.nih.gov

Royal Society for Public Health. (2017). #StatusOfMind: Social media and young people's mental health. Retrieved from https://www.rsph.org.uk

Substance Abuse and Mental Health Services Administration (SAMHSA). (2022). Behavioral health treatments and services. Retrieved from https://www.samhsa.gov

World Health Organization (WHO). (2022). Depression and other common mental disorders: Global health estimates. Retrieved from https://www.who.int

World Health Organization (WHO). (2022). Social determinants of mental health. Retrieved from https://www.who.int

Mindfulness: Being Present and In the Moment

Baer, R. A. (2003). Mindfulness training as a clinical intervention: A conceptual and empirical review. Clinical Psychology: Science and Practice, 10(2), 125-143.

Brown, K. W., & Ryan, R. M. (2003). The benefits of being present: Mindfulness and its role in psychological well-being. Journal of Personality and Social Psychology, 84(4), 822-848.

Centers for Disease Control and Prevention (CDC). (2021). Screen time and its effects on health. Retrieved from https://www.cdc.gov

Davidson, R. J., & Begley, S. (2012). The emotional life of your brain: How its unique patterns affect the way you think, feel, and live—and how you can change them. New York: Penguin Group.

Harvard Medical School. (2021). Benefits of mindfulness: Practical insights for health and well-being. Boston: Harvard Health Publishing.

Kabat-Zinn, J. (1990). Full catastrophe living: Using the wisdom of your body and mind to face stress, pain, and illness. New York: Delacorte.

Mayo Clinic. (2021). Practicing mindfulness to reduce stress and enhance focus. Retrieved from https://www.mayoclinic.org

Siegel, D. J. (2010). Mindsight: The new science of personal transformation. New York: Bantam Books.

World Health Organization (WHO). (2022). Impact of mindfulness on mental health. Retrieved from https://www.who.int

The Brain: Mastering Your Mind's Potential

Alzheimer's Association. (2021). Alzheimer's disease facts and figures. Retrieved from https://www.alz.org

American Psychological Association (APA). (2021). Stress and its effects on the brain. Retrieved from https://www.apa.org

Centers for Disease Control and Prevention (CDC). (2021). Stroke statistics and prevention. Retrieved from https://www.cdc.gov

Harvard Medical School. (2021). Understanding brain function: Insights into memory and cognition. Boston: Harvard Health Publishing.

Mayo Clinic. (2021). Brain health and lifestyle choices. Retrieved from https://www.mayoclinic.org

National Institutes of Health (NIH). (2022). Advances in neurological research: Understanding the brain's complexity. Retrieved from https://www.nih.gov

National Institute of Neurological Disorders and Stroke (NINDS). (2020). The brain's role in health and disease. Retrieved from https://www.ninds.nih.gov

World Health Organization (WHO). (2022). Neurological disorders: Global public health challenges. Retrieved from https://www.who.int

World Health Organization (WHO). (2021). Dementia and brain health: Global action plans. Retrieved from https://www.who.int

Alzheimer's Association. (2019). Lifestyle interventions for reducing dementia risk. Retrieved from https://www.alz.org

American Heart Association. (2020). The link between cardiovascular health and brain health. Retrieved from https://www.heart.org

Siegel, D. J. (2010). The mindful brain: Reflection and attunement in the cultivation of well-being. New York: W. W. Norton & Company.

Heart Health: Keeping Your Heart from Being a Time Bomb

American Heart Association (AHA). (2021). Understanding heart disease: Prevention and treatment. Retrieved from https://www.heart.org

Centers for Disease Control and Prevention (CDC). (2021). Heart disease facts and statistics. Retrieved from https://www.cdc.gov

Harvard Medical School. (2021). Heart health: Tips for prevention. Boston: Harvard Health Publishing.

Mayo Clinic. (2021). Managing heart disease through lifestyle changes. Retrieved from https://www.mayoclinic.org

National Institutes of Health (NIH). (2022). The latest research on cardiovascular diseases. Retrieved from https://www.nih.gov

World Health Organization (WHO). (2022). Global impact of cardiovascular disease. Retrieved from https://www.who.int

Cleveland Clinic. (2021). Coronary artery disease: Diagnosis and management. Retrieved from https://my.clevelandclinic.org

American College of Cardiology. (2021). Innovations in cardiac care: A focus on prevention. Journal of the American College of Cardiology, 77(8), 1032-1045. doi:10.1016/j.jacc.2021.03.004

National Heart, Lung, and Blood Institute (NHLBI). (2021). Heart-healthy living: Strategies for prevention. Retrieved from https://www.nhlbi.nih.gov

Royal Society for Public Health. (2021). The role of lifestyle in preventing cardiovascular diseases. Retrieved from https://www.rsph.org.uk

American Psychological Association (APA). (2021). The link between stress and cardiovascular health. Retrieved from https://www.apa.org

World Health Organization (WHO). (2021). The economic burden of cardiovascular diseases. Retrieved from https://www.who.int

Harvard Medical School. (2021). Innovations in heart health: The role of diet and exercise. Boston: Harvard Health Publishing.

Mayo Clinic. (2021). Early signs of heart disease: Recognizing the symptoms. Retrieved from https://www.mayoclinic.org

National Heart, Lung, and Blood Institute (NHLBI). (2021). New therapies for managing high cholesterol. Retrieved from https://www.nhlbi.nih.gov

Cleveland Clinic. (2021). Advanced imaging technologies in cardiology. Retrieved from https://my.clevelandclinic.org

World Health Organization (WHO). (2022). Cardiovascular diseases: Prevention and control strategies. Retrieved from https://www.who.int

Vital Vessels: Ensuring Healthy Circulation

American Heart Association (AHA). (2021). Understanding peripheral artery disease. Retrieved from https://www.heart.org

American Journal of Physiology. (2021). The effects of prolonged sitting on endothelial function. Journal of Applied Physiology, 131(2), 234-242. doi:10.1152/japplphysiol.00873.2021

Centers for Disease Control and Prevention (CDC). (2021). Heart disease and stroke statistics. Retrieved from https://www.cdc.gov

Harvard Medical School. (2021). Vascular health: Keeping your arteries and veins in top condition. Boston: Harvard Health Publishing.

Mayo Clinic. (2021). Peripheral artery disease: Causes and prevention. Retrieved from https://www.mayoclinic.org

National Institutes of Health (NIH). (2022). Advances in circulatory system research. Retrieved from https://www.nih.gov

Society for Vascular Surgery. (2021). Understanding varicose veins and treatments. Retrieved from https://www.vascular.org

World Health Organization (WHO). (2022). The global burden of vascular diseases. Retrieved from https://www.who.int

American College of Cardiology. (2021). The role of lifestyle in preventing circulatory diseases. Journal of the American College of Cardiology, 78(4), 389-401. doi:10.1016/j.jacc.2021.05.022

National Heart, Lung, and Blood Institute (NHLBI). (2021). Managing cholesterol for circulatory health. Retrieved from https://www.nhlbi.nih.gov

Cleveland Clinic. (2021). Comprehensive guide to deep vein thrombosis (DVT). Retrieved from https://my.clevelandclinic.org

American Vascular Association. (2021). Promoting vein health: Tips and treatments. Retrieved from https://vascular.org

World Health Organization (WHO). (2021). Global action plans for noncommunicable diseases. Retrieved from https://www.who.int

Harvard Medical School. (2021). The science of blood circulation. Boston: Harvard Health Publishing.

Centers for Disease Control and Prevention (CDC). (2022). Lifestyle changes for better vascular health. Retrieved from https://www.cdc.gov

Mayo Clinic. (2021). Tips for preventing blood clots and promoting circulation. Retrieved from https://www.mayoclinic.org

American Psychological Association (APA). (2021). The psychological effects of circulatory health conditions. Retrieved from https://www.apa.org

Royal Society for Public Health. (2021). Physical activity and its impact on vascular health. Retrieved from https://www.rsph.org.uk

National Institute on Aging (NIA). (2022). Aging and the circulatory system. Retrieved from https://www.nia.nih.gov

Breaking Free of Vices – You Can Be a Healthier You

American Psychological Association (APA). (2021). Addiction and behavior: Understanding the cycles. Retrieved from https://www.apa.org

Centers for Disease Control and Prevention (CDC). (2021). Alcohol and public health: Statistics and impact. Retrieved from https://www.cdc.gov

Centers for Disease Control and Prevention (CDC). (2021). Smoking and tobacco use: Key facts. Retrieved from https://www.cdc.gov

Harvard Medical School. (2021). Strategies for overcoming addiction: A medical perspective. Boston: Harvard Health Publishing.

Mayo Clinic. (2021). Managing substance abuse and dependencies. Retrieved from https://www.mayoclinic.org

National Institute on Drug Abuse (NIDA). (2021). The science of addiction: How substances affect the brain. Retrieved from https://www.drugabuse.gov

National Institute on Alcohol Abuse and Alcoholism (NIAAA). (2021). Alcohol use disorder: Symptoms and treatment. Retrieved from https://www.niaaa.nih.gov

Royal Society for Public Health. (2021). Social factors and their role in addiction recovery. Retrieved from https://www.rsph.org.uk

Substance Abuse and Mental Health Services Administration (SAMHSA). (2022). Resources for overcoming substance abuse. Retrieved from https://www.samhsa.gov

World Health Organization (WHO). (2022). Global statistics on alcohol and tobacco use. Retrieved from https://www.who.int

American Cancer Society. (2021). Smoking and its link to cancer: A comprehensive review. Retrieved from https://www.cancer.org

American Heart Association (AHA). (2021). Cardiovascular risks associated with smoking and drinking. Retrieved from https://www.heart.org

Harvard Medical School. (2021). Mindfulness and addiction recovery: Clinical insights. Boston: Harvard Health Publishing.

National Institute of Mental Health (NIMH). (2021). The role of mental health in overcoming addiction. Retrieved from https://www.nimh.nih.gov

Cleveland Clinic. (2021). Behavioral therapy and addiction treatment. Retrieved from https://my.clevelandclinic.org

World Health Organization (WHO). (2022). Strategies for global substance abuse prevention. Retrieved from https://www.who.int

National Institutes of Health (NIH). (2022). Advances in addiction recovery research. Retrieved from https://www.nih.gov

The Power of Prevention: Building a Healthier Tomorrow

American Heart Association (AHA). (2021). Preventing heart disease: A guide to healthy living. Retrieved from https://www.heart.org

American Psychological Association (APA). (2021). The role of mental health in preventative care. Retrieved from https://www.apa.org

Centers for Disease Control and Prevention (CDC). (2021). Chronic diseases in America: Statistics and prevention. Retrieved from https://www.cdc.gov

Centers for Disease Control and Prevention (CDC). (2021). Vaccination schedules for children and adults. Retrieved from https://www.cdc.gov/vaccines

Harvard Medical School. (2021). Nutrition and disease prevention: Insights into healthy living. Boston: Harvard Health Publishing.

Mayo Clinic. (2021). Screening and early detection for chronic diseases. Retrieved from https://www.mayoclinic.org

National Institutes of Health (NIH). (2022). Advances in preventative medicine: Reducing risks through lifestyle changes. Retrieved from https://www.nih.gov

World Health Organization (WHO). (2022). Global strategies for chronic disease prevention. Retrieved from https://www.who.int

World Health Organization (WHO). (2021). The role of vaccinations in public health. Retrieved from https://www.who.int

American Cancer Society. (2021). Early detection and prevention of cancer: A statistical analysis. Retrieved from https://www.cancer.org

National Cancer Institute (NCI). (2021). Understanding genetic risks in cancer prevention. Retrieved from https://www.cancer.gov

Cleveland Clinic. (2021). The importance of regular check-ups for early disease detection. Retrieved from https://my.clevelandclinic.org

Royal Society for Public Health. (2021). The impact of lifestyle choices on chronic disease prevention. Retrieved from https://www.rsph.org.uk

Harvard Medical School. (2021). The benefits of exercise on cardiovascular health. Boston: Harvard Health Publishing.

National Institute of Mental Health (NIMH). (2021). Addressing mental health in preventive care strategies. Retrieved from https://www.nimh.nih.gov

American Academy of Pediatrics. (2021). Vaccinations and children's health: A comprehensive guide. Retrieved from https://www.aap.org

Substance Abuse and Mental Health Services Administration (SAMHSA). (2022). Behavioral health and its role in prevention. Retrieved from https://www.samhsa.gov

World Health Organization (WHO). (2022). Environmental factors in preventative health: Addressing air and water quality. Retrieved from https://www.who.int

National Heart, Lung, and Blood Institute (NHLBI). (2021). Reducing risks through preventive cardiovascular care. Retrieved from https://www.nhlbi.nih.gov

U.S. Preventive Services Task Force. (2021). Guidelines for screening and prevention. Retrieved from https://www.uspreventiveservicestaskforce.org

Health for All Women: Addressing Our Unique Needs and Maintaining Long-Term Wellness

American Academy of Pediatrics. (2021). Guidelines on child health. Retrieved from https://www.aap.org

American Cancer Society. (2021). Breast cancer facts and figures. Retrieved from https://www.cancer.org

American Heart Association. (2021). Cardiovascular disease in women: Key statistics. Retrieved from https://www.heart.org

American Sexual Health Association. (2021). Women and STIs: Key facts. Retrieved from https://www.ashasexualhealth.org

Centers for Disease Control and Prevention (CDC). (2021). Women's health: Overview and priorities. Retrieved from https://www.cdc.gov

Cleveland Clinic. (2021). Hormonal changes during menopause: What to expect. Retrieved from https://my.clevelandclinic.org

Harvard Medical School. (2021). Women's health: Advancing care and research. Boston: Harvard Health Publishing.

Mayo Clinic. (2021). Preventive health screenings for women. Retrieved from https://www.mayoclinic.org

Mayo Clinic. (2021). Osteoporosis prevention: Calcium and vitamin D intake. Retrieved from https://www.mayoclinic.org

National Institutes of Health (NIH). (2022). Understanding menopause: Research and treatment. Retrieved from https://www.nih.gov

National Institute of Mental Health (NIMH). (2021). Mental health and hormonal influences in women. Retrieved from https://www.nimh.nih.gov

National Osteoporosis Foundation. (2021). Understanding bone health: Preventing fractures. Retrieved from https://www.nof.org

Substance Abuse and Mental Health Services Administration (SAMHSA). (2022). Behavioral health and women: Addressing unique challenges. Retrieved from https://www.samhsa.gov

World Health Organization (WHO). (2022). Women's health and well-being: Global perspectives. Retrieved from https://www.who.int

World Health Organization (WHO). (2022). Preventing cervical cancer: The role of HPV vaccinations. Retrieved from https://www.who.int

U.S. Preventive Services Task Force. (2021). Guidelines for women's health screenings. Retrieved from https://www.uspreventiveservicestaskforce.org

Health for All Men: Recognizing the Barriers that Keep US from Seeking Help

American Cancer Society. (2021). Prostate cancer statistics and prevention. Retrieved from https://www.cancer.org

American Heart Association (AHA). (2021). Cardiovascular health in men: Risk factors and prevention. Retrieved from https://www.heart.org

Centers for Disease Control and Prevention (CDC). (2021). Men's health statistics and prevention strategies. Retrieved from https://www.cdc.gov

Cleveland Clinic. (2021). Comprehensive guide to prostate health. Retrieved from https://my.clevelandclinic.org

Harvard Medical School. (2021). The role of testosterone in men's health. Boston: Harvard Health Publishing.

Mayo Clinic. (2021). Erectile dysfunction: Causes, treatments, and prevention. Retrieved from https://www.mayoclinic.org

National Institute of Diabetes and Digestive and Kidney Diseases (NIDDK). (2021). Diabetes and men: Risk factors and management. Retrieved from https://www.niddk.nih.gov

National Institutes of Health (NIH). (2022). Advances in men's health research. Retrieved from https://www.nih.gov

National Institute of Mental Health (NIMH). (2021). Men's mental health: Addressing stigma and access to care. Retrieved from https://www.nimh.nih.gov

Royal Society for Public Health. (2021). Social determinants of men's health: Insights and interventions. Retrieved from https://www.rsph.org.uk

Substance Abuse and Mental Health Services Administration (SAMHSA). (2022). Mental health resources for men. Retrieved from https://www.samhsa.gov

World Health Organization (WHO). (2022). Global strategies for addressing men's health disparities. Retrieved from https://www.who.int

Harvard Medical School. (2021). Physical activity and its benefits for men's health. Boston: Harvard Health Publishing.

American Urological Association. (2021). Guidelines for managing benign prostatic hyperplasia. Retrieved from https://www.auanet.org

American Psychological Association (APA). (2021). Stress and its impact on men's health. Retrieved from https://www.apa.org

National Cancer Institute (NCI). (2021). Understanding the genetic risk factors in men's cancers. Retrieved from https://www.cancer.gov

Mayo Clinic. (2021). Supplements for prostate health: Evidence and recommendations. Retrieved from https://www.mayoclinic.org

Harvard Medical School. (2021). Enhancing sexual health through lifestyle changes. Boston: Harvard Health Publishing.

Centers for Disease Control and Prevention (CDC). (2021). Preventative screenings for men by age. Retrieved from https://www.cdc.gov

The Next Generation: Giving Our Children a Healthy Start on a Healthy Life

American Academy of Pediatrics (AAP). (2021). Guidelines on pediatric health care. Retrieved from https://www.aap.org

American Psychological Association (APA). (2021). Childhood mental health: Understanding anxiety and depression. Retrieved from https://www.apa.org

Centers for Disease Control and Prevention (CDC). (2021). Vaccination schedules for children and adolescents. Retrieved from https://www.cdc.gov

Centers for Disease Control and Prevention (CDC). (2021). Screen time recommendations for children. Retrieved from https://www.cdc.gov

Cleveland Clinic. (2021). Managing childhood asthma: Guidelines and tips. Retrieved from https://my.clevelandclinic.org

Harvard Medical School. (2021). The importance of play in child development. Boston: Harvard Health Publishing.

Mayo Clinic. (2021). Nutritional guidelines for children. Retrieved from https://www.mayoclinic.org

National Institutes of Health (NIH). (2022). Advances in pediatric care and research. Retrieved from https://www.nih.gov

National Institute of Mental Health (NIMH). (2021). Mental health in children: Early detection and prevention. Retrieved from https://www.nimh.nih.gov

Royal Society for Public Health (RSPH). (2021). The impact of social media on children's mental health. Retrieved from https://www.rsph.org.uk

Substance Abuse and Mental Health Services Administration (SAMHSA).

(2022). Resources for addressing childhood mental health issues. Retrieved from https://www.samhsa.gov

World Health Organization (WHO). (2022). Global strategies for improving child health outcomes. Retrieved from https://www.who.int

World Health Organization (WHO). (2022). Environmental impacts on pediatric health. Retrieved from https://www.who.int

Harvard Medical School. (2021). The role of early childhood education in cognitive development. Boston: Harvard Health Publishing.

American Lung Association. (2021). Preventing and managing childhood respiratory illnesses. Retrieved from https://www.lung.org

American Academy of Pediatrics (AAP). (2021). The importance of developmental screenings in pediatrics. Retrieved from https://www.aap.org

National Institute on Drug Abuse (NIDA). (2021). Preventing substance abuse among youth. Retrieved from https://www.drugabuse.gov

American Heart Association (AHA). (2021). Encouraging physical activity in children to prevent heart disease. Retrieved from https://www.heart.org

National Institute of Diabetes and Digestive and Kidney Diseases (NIDDK). (2021). Addressing childhood obesity: Tips for families. Retrieved from https://www.niddk.nih.gov

Centers for Disease Control and Prevention (CDC). (2022). Recognizing and managing common childhood illnesses. Retrieved from https://www.cdc.gov

Ratey, J. (2008). *Spark: The Revolutionary New Science of Exercise and the Brain*. Little, Brown Spark.

Ornish, D. (2007). *The Spectrum: A Scientifically Proven Program to Feel Better, Live Longer, Lose Weight, and Gain Health*. Ballantine Books.

Lustig, R. H. (2012). *Fat Chance: Beating the Odds Against Sugar, Processed Food, Obesity, and Disease*. Hudson Street Press.

Hyman, M. (2012). *The Blood Sugar Solution: The UltraHealthy Program for Losing Weight, Preventing Disease, and Feeling Great Now!*. Little, Brown.

Sapolsky, R. M. (2004). *Why Zebras Don't Get Ulcers: The Acclaimed Guide to Stress, Stress-Related Diseases, and Coping*. Henry Holt and Company.

Ratey, J. J., & Hagerman, E. (2008). *Spark: The Revolutionary New Science of Exercise and the Brain*. Little, Brown Spark.

Buettner, D. (2023). *The Blue Zones Secrets for Living Longer: Lessons From the Healthiest Places on Earth*. National Geographic.

National Academies of Sciences, Engineering, and Medicine. (2017). *The Health Effects of Cannabis and Cannabinoids: The Current State of Evidence and Recommendations for Research*. The National Academies Press. https://doi.org/10.17226/24625

Centers for Medicare & Medicaid Services. (2021). *National Health Expenditure Data*. https://www.cms.gov/Research-Statistics-Data-and-Systems/Statistics-Trends-and-Reports/NationalHealthExpendData

ABOUT THE AUTHORS

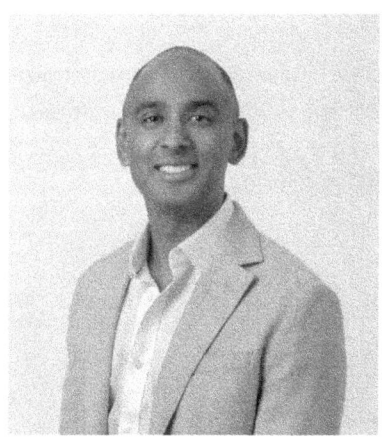

Dr. Raja Ramaswamy is a physician, health columnist, and author focused on making medicine more practical and empowering. Born and raised in Anderson, Indiana, he writes regularly on health and public policy, contributes to major media outlets, and speaks nationally on innovation in patient care and wellness. He is deeply committed to advancing health equity and making high-quality care accessible to all communities.

Raja is a graduate of Emory University and Chicago Medical School. He lives in Carmel, Indiana with his wife, Hillary, and their two children. In addition to his clinical work, he is a vocal advocate for preventive care, health literacy, and restoring trust in the patient-physician relationship.

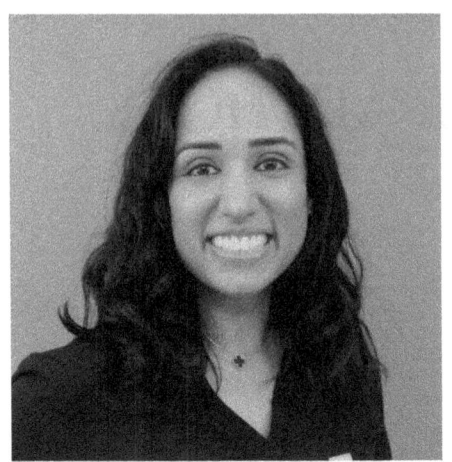

Dr. Rani Ramaswamy is an OB-GYN and health advocate dedicated to advancing women's health through compassionate, evidence-based, and culturally sensitive care. Her clinical work focuses on reproductive health, maternal wellness, and preventive medicine, with a strong emphasis on patient education and empowerment.

She is a graduate of Chicago Medical School. Rani lives in Carmel, Indiana with her husband, Nirdhar, and their three children. Passionate about health equity and community engagement, she continues to champion access to comprehensive, personalized care for women at every stage of life.

www.ingramcontent.com/pod-product-compliance
Lightning Source LLC
Chambersburg PA
CBHW020455030426
42337CB00011B/126